The Conquest of Bacteria

The Conquest of Bacteria

From Salvarsan to Sulphapyridine

by

FRANK SHERWOOD TAYLOR

Foreword by

HENRY E. SIGERIST

Essay Index Reprint Series

BOOKS FOR LIBRARIES PRESS

FREEPORT, NEW YORK

INTERNATIONAL STANDARD BOOK NUMBER:
0-8369-2375-8

LIBRARY OF CONGRESS CATALOG CARD NUMBER:
78-142705

PRINTED IN THE UNITED STATES OF AMERICA

FOREWORD

The Greeks made the two greatest discoveries that could be made in medicine. They found that disease is a natural process, not basically different from normal or physiological processes. They discovered, in addition, that the human body possesses an innate healing power which tends to overcome lesions and to restore the balanced condition which they considered health.

These views directed their actions. The physician's task in treating a disease was to support and aid the healing power of nature and to avoid any measure that could possibly counteract it. They did this by regulating the patient's diet and entire mode of living, by enhancing the action of foods with drugs, and they found that in certain cases surgery could accelerate the healing process.

For over two thousand years very little progress was made in the treatment of diseases. Medical science advanced. The structure of the body became intimately known, the functions of the organs were studied in health and disease, disease entities were established, and the causes of many, particularly of infectious diseases, were elucidated. This was very important because it made it possible to protect man against many diseases. But when it came to the treatment of an ailment, the physician was almost as helpless as he had been two thousand years before, and he could not do much more than follow the old Hippocratic principles.

Throughout history drugs were given in great quantities and in odd combinations. The patient's desire for more than verbal advice forced the physician to act, and so he prescribed purgatives and vomitives that evacuated faulty matters or remedies that alleviated the sick man's symptoms. Pharmacology was an empirical science. A drug given because experience taught that it helped, and the accumulated experience of millenia was not to be despised. Mercury did cure syphilis, and quinine malaria in some mysterious ways. Digitalis did help in heart diseases and opium relieved pain.

In the second half of the 19th century pharmacology became an experimental science closely connected with physiology. It studied the action of chemical compounds on the normal and sick organism and was able to produce many valuable drugs. Vitamins and hormones enabled man to prevent and cure a number of deficiency and other diseases. In recent years such deadly diseases as pernicious anemia and diabetes could be treated successfully. Nevertheless the hero of therapy was still the surgeon. He could save a man's life in a way that was apparent to all. If a patient suffering from an internal disease recovered, you usually could not tell how much credit was due to the physician and how much to nature's healing power.

The situation has changed since Paul Ehrlich inaugurated modern chemotherapy. The great expectations raised by his discovery of Salvarsan in 1910 were somewhat disappointed, and it was felt for a while that chemotherapy had reached a dead end. The new drugs were highly successful in the treatment of diseases caused by a certain group of protozoa but had no effect on bacteria. Then came Domagk and sulphanilamide. This was in 1935, only yesterday. Today we can already say that these new drugs have revolutionized medicine, and we can be grateful that there was time enough to gain experience with them before the war broke out.

I like Mr. Taylor's book very much because it presents the story of chemotherapy in terms which are the more impressive because they are simple and sober. This is the best type of popular book on a scientific subject, and it should be most welcome to the thousands of people who have read accounts of the new miracle drugs in the newspapers and would like to know what it is all about.

Scientific research of less than half a century has shown that chemical compounds can cure many diseases caused not only by trypanosomes but also by bacteria. There is no doubt that more drugs can be found that will destroy more bacteria, and we are justified in hoping that chemotherapy may also cure diseases that are caused by a filterable virus. If our hopes are to be fulfilled, we must have more and more research, and Mr. Taylor ends his book with a strong and well motivated plea for increased public support of research.

HENRY E. SIGERIST

The Johns Hopkins Institute of the
History of Medicine.

CONTENTS

CONTENTS

CHAPTER VI

CHAPTER VII

CHAPTER VIII

CHAPTER IX

CHAPTER X

INTRODUCTION

DURING the last few years a new way of treating certain common and serious diseases has come into prominence. This new weapon in the physician's armoury is known as Chemotherapy, and deserves a high place among modern discoveries inasmuch as it has already saved thousands of lives and promises to save many thousands more. It is applicable only to those diseases which are caused by a living parasite—whether protozoon, bacterium, or virus-particle—multiplying within the body; for it consists of administering a drug which is designed to bring about the death of these parasites without harm to their host.

Drugs are the oldest recourse of the physician, and even today something-out-of-a-medicine-bottle is the only treatment in which a large section of the public has real confidence. It is very hard indeed to persuade a man who is not already prostrate with disease to alter his food or drink or the quantity of exercise he takes, but he will gladly take any quantity of medicine. But until a few years ago none of the actual bacterial diseases, e.g. pneumonia, typhoid fever, blood-poisoning, could be radically cured by any kind of medicine. No

drug could strike at the root of the trouble — the
bacterium in the tissues — and so remove the
cause of the disease and bring it to an abrupt
close. The drugs which the doctor prescribed were
designed to alleviate symptoms, or to increase or
diminish some bodily function. Thus aspirin
would alleviate pain, sulphonal would bring sleep,
codeine would repress a cough, but the curing of
the disease was done by the intimate mechanism
of the patient's own body, aided perhaps by anti-
toxins or sera, elaborated — none knew how —
in the body of an animal.

Yet there were exceptions to this rule, for two
diseases were radically influenced by drugs and
could be cured by them, despite the fact that
without their aid patients recovered from them
very slowly or not at all. These were malarial
fever and syphilis. In the sixteenth century it was
found that mercury compounds would cure syphilis — a disease which seemed never to cure itself spontaneously; in the seventeenth century
cinchona bark — the active principle of which
is quinine — was found to be very successful in
curing malaria. Yet between this early period
and the twentieth century there were no further
additions to these remedies. This discovery that
a great number of diseases were due to the invasion of the body by living germs led at once to
amazing progress towards the prevention of disease — in civilized countries, at least. Yet this
progress must not be exaggerated, for to-day,
sixty years after the general acceptance of the

germ-theory, the world has not found it practically possible to prevent the majority of germ-diseases. Malaria, plague, cholera, typhoid, leprosy, sleeping-sickness, ravage the tropics, while at home tuberculosis, various types of septic conditions, pneumonia, meningitis, whooping cough, measles, still claim their annual quota of victims. For these diseases, then, which we cannot or will not prevent, there is urgent need for a means of cure. Up to forty years ago the physician could do little to aid those who suffered from such diseases. His chief recourse was what we may call good nursing, that is to say, the provision of surroundings and conditions in which the body should be best able to do its own repairs.

The discovery of serum-therapy and anti-toxins has done something toward the cure of these diseases; but, save in one or two brilliant instances, notably that of diphtheria, they have proved to be but uncertain aids.

During the last thirty years, and especially during the last five, the method of chemotherapy has become an important and effective means of combating some of these diseases. In 1907 Ehrlich succeeded in finding a synthetic drug, atoxyl, which would cure many cases of sleeping-sickness by killing the parasites in the patient's blood; in 1910 he revolutionized the treatment of syphilis by his famous drug '606.' Between this date and 1935, research has brought into use drugs capable of combating every form of tropical disease. The treatment of one of these alone — I refer to kala-azar, a disease of which few people have even heard — has saved some three hundred thousand lives.

The drugs in use before 1935 were effective only against protozoa — the minute animal parasites which cause most of the tropical diseases — and none of them had the power of destroying bacteria, invasion by which is the cause of most of the germ-diseases common in temperate climates. Such diseases include blood-poisoning, numerous septic conditions, pneumonia, meningitis, tuberculosis, and many others. In 1935, however, Domagk announced the discovery of a new drug — prontosil — which had spectacular effects on diseases caused by that deadly and hitherto unassailable bacterium, the β-hæmolytic streptococcus. This drug was the first of a new group, termed the sulphonamide drugs, the most important of which proved to be a fairly simple chemical compound, sulphanilamide. This new group wrought marvels in the treatment of erysipelas, septic wounds, cellulitis, septicæmia, and above all the dreaded puerperal fever, which, in this country alone, yearly killed thousands of mothers. Finally, in 1938, appeared the amazing compound M and B 693 (dagenan or sulphapyridine) which is capable of causing the destruction in our bodies not only of the β-hæmolytic streptococcus, but also of the pneumococcus, the meningococcus, and the gonococcus, so completely revolutionizing the treatment not only of the diseases named above, but also of pneumonia, cerebrospinal meningitis, gonorrhœa, and several other less well-known diseases.

It is an understatement to say that three-quarters of those who formerly died from these diseases can now be saved. And when we reflect that in this country no less than twelve thousand people died every year of lobar pneumonia, the gigantic significance of this work becomes apparent. This benefit to humanity did not fall from heaven: it was the result of a long, skilled, and deliberate research. Not a penny of public money was expended on this work, which was almost entirely carried out by commercial firms, whose business it is to sell drugs and make a profit. Is this a satisfactory state of affairs? The task of chemotherapy is not completed, for there are a great many germ-diseases for which no remedy is known. Tuberculosis is the outstanding example. The *Mycobacterium tuberculosis* which causes it is not affected by the new drugs. Yet it is an organism closely similar to those which causes the diseases we have conquered in this fashion and there is no reason whatever to suppose that a chemotherapeutic remedy for it cannot be found. It is even possible that this remedy is now lying on the organic chemist's shelves, as sulphanilamide lay for a quarter of a century before its powers were known. But that remedy will be found only by lengthy and painstaking research. That research will be done; but the rate at which it will be done, and also the time which will elapse before it is completed, will depend closely upon the quantity of money spent upon it.

Is this money to be the amount that fine-chemical firms can profitably allocate to research, or is it to be found by the government — that is, by you and me? A tiny beginning has been made, but this is far from enough.

My brother, gassed in the war of 1914-1918, and dying of tuberculosis of the larynx, wrote on a piece of paper — for he could not speak — 'This is what modern science has done for me.' The world is again at war and is spending perhaps some twenty millions a day on weapons of death and defenses against them. Yet we will not spend five thousand dollars a day in the hope of winning a permanent victory over the grim wolf who was with us when Egypt warred with Babylon, who each year carries off tens of thousands of men, and who, if we help not ourselves, will still be slaying us when the present war is but a dusty item in the historian's count of crime and its reward.

CHAPTER I

BACTERIA AND DISEASE

Historical — The germ theory today — Protozoa
— Bacteria — Virus particles — Transmis-
sion of infections — Preventive medicine
— Its limitations.

L ONG ago, perhaps indeed as soon as there
arose the idea of the existence of specific diseases, physicians recognized a group of ailments
which they termed *fevers* — meaning thereby
conditions in which the patient's body appeared
hotter than it did when he was in health. Early
physicians had no thermometers to tell them of a
rise in the patient's temperature, and even after
adequate instruments had been perfected by Roe-
mer, Fahrenheit, and others, at the beginning of
the eighteenth century, they were not brought into
medical practice. It was not indeed until the eighteen-sixties that doctors began to take their patient's temperatures. But the good physician is a
keen observer, and some of the scientific aids he
lacked were replaced by a shrewd eye and sensitive hand. We may have little doubt, then, that
even a mild degree of fever was detected by the
doctor's hand — though no doubt patients, house-

wives, and even nurses, went much astray.

The classification of fevers was a difficult task. Today the bacteriologist can settle points of doubt, but in the early nineteenth century diseases could only be classified by their outwardly manifest symptoms. Most of the more obvious diseases were, however, recognized, among them malaria — at that date prevalent in England, — typhoid fever (apt to be confused with the very different typhus), cholera, small-pox, scarlet fever, measles, pneumonia and, of course, the venereal diseases. It could not escape the observation of medical men that some of these diseases were epidemic. An epidemic disease is one, of which at times very few cases are to found, but which occasionally breaks out and affects an increasing number of people until a peak-point of prevalence is reached, after which the number of cases once more declines until the disease nearly disappears. Other fevers seemed to be endemic; that is to say, cases of them were always to be found in numbers which did not vary greatly; others again partook of both characters.

Today we naturally think of these diseases as infections, because we have been brought up in a world which educates its citizens, in school and also by newspapers and advertisements, to believe in the dangers of infection. In the eighteen-fifties the world thought very differently. The medical men of the eighteen-fifties were familiar with great epidemics of typhoid fever and cholera destroying their patients by thousands. They saw ty-

phoid fever or cholera attacking people who had
not come within hailing distance of another case,
and naturally were much puzzled as to what the
cause of the disease might be. We know today
that the cause was typhoid or cholera bacteria
which had found their way in a typhoid or cholera patient's excreta to the patient's drinking-
water — usually unfiltered river or shallow well-
water. The idea that typhoid fever and cholera
might arise from polluted water occurred but
rarely to the men of the time, and when it was
suggested it did not seem plausible, for everyone
knew that hundreds of thousands of folk drank
little else but polluted water and remained quite
healthy. The general view was that epidemic diseases were spread by non-living vapors or gases,
arising from marshy ground, decaying organic
matter, or what-not. These were called miasmas,
putrid exhalations, putrescent streams, etc. It was
this theory that gave Florence Nightingale her
passionate belief in fresh air, a belief which has
spread through a whole civilized world and is
held with a largely irrational fervor. At this
period there was indeed much doubt as to whether any, and if so which, diseases were conveyed
from the sick to the healthy. Many medical men
believed that some general subtle alteration of the
air or some other external conditions caused the
epidemics, and very few would have supposed
such a disease as tuberculosis to be transmitted
from the diseased to the healthy.

In the eighteen-sixties, then, the cause of the

majority of diseases was unknown. Theories, of course, abounded, as they always do when knowledge is scarce. Some medical men even held the true theory of a living contagion; but since they could advance no better reasons than the holders of other theories, their views carried no conviction. It was accepted that there was some connection between some kinds of dirt and some kinds of disease, for populations which lived in insanitary places suffered more from fevers than did those who lived in fairly clean places; but the exact nature of this connection remained unproven and largely unsuspected until Louis Pasteur, between 1860 and 1880, gradually brought it to light, and so conferred on the human race enormously the greatest material benefit which it has yet received.

Scientific problems are not solved by the sudden appearance of a genius. Had Pasteur been born in the sixteenth century he could not have fathomed the nature of disease, for, in the chaos of scientific ignorance which then prevailed, he could have found no solid ground to stand on. Even in 1860 he could hardly have succeeded in a frontal attack on the problem of disease, the solution of which, like most great scientific discoveries, resulted from the following up of a train of thought and experiment which started with quite a different purpose. Pasteur started his series of researches by trying to improve beer, and ended by causing the greatest revolution in the world's health that has ever been or is likely to be. Pasteur was a research chemist not a medical

man.   As a very young man he carried out a brilliant research on the asymmetry of certain crys-
tals, from which has sprung a whole department
of science which we now call stereochemistry.   He
might have continued these rather academic researches had it not chanced that his first important post was at Lille, in a district where brew-
ing and the fermentation of mash for making spir-
its were staple industries.   Pasteur throughout his
life was a very practical person.   He did his work
with the constant object of benefiting humanity
in general and France in particular by improving manufactures, commerce, or health.   Accordingly, he began to investigate the troubles of the
brewer.   Beer is subject to 'diseases'; during its
manufacture something may unaccountably go
wrong, leading to the production of an ill-flav-
ored or even undrinkable brew.   Pasteur made a
study of fermentation, the process by which a
weak sugary solution, such as the infusion of
malt from which beer is brewed, is converted into carbon dioxide and alcohol.   It was, of course,
well known that a living organism, yeast, always
appeared and multiplied greatly in quantity,
when wort fermented into beer.   The view of the
time, sponsored by the great Baron Liebig —
then a formidable authority — was that the
growth of the yeast was not an essential feature
of the process, but a minor incident, and that
fermentation was a simple chemical reaction by
which glucose was changed to carbon dioxide and
alcohol under the influence of a non-living 'fer-

ment' independent of the living yeast cells. The result of Pasteur's work was the proof that there was no fermentation without yeast and that if a solution fermented without yeast being intentionally added, it did so as the result of living yeast particles entering it from the air, in which they had been floating. He established, to his own satisfaction at least, that living yeast was a necessary link in the chain of events which transformed sugar to alcohol. Now the souring of milk is very like fermentation, and so is the putrefaction or 'going bad' of an animal liquid such as broth. He saw that all these phenomena were closely connected, and proved by several years of unassailable experiment that putrefaction would not take place without the co-operation of living organisms. These organisms he showed were ubiquitous, and they were always present in the air as dust. He proved that liquids such as broth, milk, urine, etc., which had been boiled so as to kill all organisms, would not putrefy in contact with air which had been filtered from dust or strongly heated. By 1864 Pasteur had proved to the satisfaction of the more reasonable part, but not the whole, of the scientific world that putrefaction did not occur except as a result of the presence of living 'germs' and their rapid multiplication; and that these 'germs' were not generated in the process of putrefaction, but were the offspring of other germs introduced from without. This discovery of the nature of putrefaction and the virtual disproof of spontaneous generation settled two questions which had stood in doubt since the days of the first Greek philosophers; yet Pasteur was on the threshold of a discovery still greater — the nature of contagious disease. But he was not a medical man and it would not have been natural to him to attempt to investigate this field directly, and, in fact, he approached it only through a study of the diseases of animals.

But, meanwhile, Pasteur's hint was taken up by a great surgeon, Joseph Lister. He had been studying the nature of surgical sepsis. In those days, all surgical wounds became septic — that is to say, they became inflamed and exuded a fluid called pus, which in some cases had an odor of putrefaction. At the same time, the patient developed, as a rule, some degree of fever. If the sepsis was very widespread, and especially if the pus was not allowed to drain freely from the wound, the patient became gravely ill and often died. Just under half of Lister's amputation cases died directly or indirectly from this cause, and a mortality of four in five was not uncommon in less skilful hands. Lister had come to the conclusion that a wound became septic because of the putrefaction of the fluids in and about it. But what was putrefaction and how could it be prevented? In 1865 a colleague called his attention to Pasteur's work. Lister argued that if, as Pasteur would seem to have proved, putrefaction resulted from living germs floating in the air and adherent to all ordinary objects, he could prevent the putrefaction of a wound by destroying the germs around the wound and excluding the others from entering. Lister looked at the matter from the point of view of surgery rather than biology. He was not specially concerned to know what sort of creatures these 'germs' might be; for he knew all that he needed to know, that they caused sepsis and that he was able to kill them by the action of heat and certain chemicals.

So he sterilized instruments and dressings and covered the wound with carbolic acid. His success was phenomenal, and, rather slowly, the surgical world was driven to adopt his methods. Lister's elasticity of mind was remarkable. He altered his methods continually, ever keeping in mind the one purpose of destroying and excluding living germs, and so in the years between 1865 and 1887 built up the technique of modern surgery.

This work, one might think, was a very plain hint that disease might be due to 'germs' — for here was a man avowedly excluding germs and thereby preventing some of the worst of diseases — hospital gangrene and blood-poisoning. But the men of the time did not see the connection, and it was Pasteur who carried on the work. In the year 1865 he was asked to investigate a disease of silkworms, which was ruining the exceedingly important silk-industry of France. His studies of fermentation and the 'diseases' of beer and wine set his thoughts in the right direction and he proved that the disease was caused by micro-

scopic parasites which multiplied within the
silkworms' bodies and were transferred from one
silkworm to another, so spreading the disease.
Here was another plain hint; but it was not taken.
The analogy between diseases of silkworms and
diseases of man was not close enough to be
grasped by the minds of the generality of scien-
tists and medical men; and Pasteur himself seems
hardly to have envisaged its possibilities.   In
1868, moreover, he suffered a severe illness which
interrupted his work, and when he had recovered sufficiently to take up research once more,
he returned to his first interest, that of fermentation, and for fourteen years he made no further
investigations of disease.   In 1863-1868 Davaine
investigated the disease of anthrax which affects
both cattle and men.   He actually saw anthrax
bacilli in the blood of infected animals and really
proved them to be the cause of the disease.   In
1873 Obermeier saw minute parasites in the blood
of a patient suffering from relapsing fever.   None
of this attracted much interest, and it was the researches of Robert Koch, who founded the practical technique of bacteriology, and those of Pasteur on inoculation of animals against chicken
cholera and anthrax, which converted the world
to the germ-theory.   In 1876 Koch made studies
of anthrax and showed how bacteria could be
isolated, cultured and stained; and in 1878 he
published a book on the infection of wounds,
showing the nature of the organisms which infected them — the 'germs' which had been suc-

cessfully combated by Lister, despite his lack of knowledge of their exact nature. The year 1880, then, may be taken to mark the period when the world began to be aware that many diseases were caused by the multiplication of microscopic parasites within the bodies of the animals affected. This idea, which we may call the germ-theory of disease, made rapid progress; between 1880 and 1900 the parasites which caused most of the common diseases were recognized, grown in pure culture, and described.

At this stage let us leave the history of the germ-theory and take stock of our present beliefs about parasites and disease.

It has been proved, without any doubt, that a large class of diseases is the result of the presence and multiplication of living organisms in the body of the man or animal affected. Each species of organism produces characteristic symptoms, though the manifestation of them may vary according to the part of the body infected. Thus the characteristic effect of the bacterium we call *streptococcus pneumoniæ* (or the *pneumococcus*) is to invade and congest the lung-substance, so causing the disease we call lobar pneumonia; but, on rare occasions, it may infect the lining membranes of the brain and so cause pneumococcal meningitis. Generally speaking then, the patient's symptoms depend both on the species of organism which attacks him and the site of its attack.

The parasite does not damage the body by its mere presence, but by its products. The microscopic parasites which cause disease produce non-living poisons or toxins. Thus, if we grow certain disease-bacteria in a nutrient liquid, and then filter that liquid through porous pottery so as to remove all the bacteria from it, the liquid is found to be poisonous. If this liquid is injected into an animal, it is capable of producing in the animal some of the symptoms of the disease associated with the bacteria in question; yet the liquid will not produce the disease itself — for this the living bacteria are required.

As an example we may take the disease of diphtheria, which has been known for about a century. The obvious seat of the trouble is the patient's throat, where there forms an adherent 'false membrane.' But the patient at the same time becomes gravely ill and is more likely to die from the failure of his heart than from suffocation due to the 'membrane' blocking the air-passages. In 1883 it was shown that diphtheria was the result of a bacterium, the Klebs-Loeffler bacillus (*Corynebacterium diphtheriæ*), which grew in the patient's throat and without which no case of diphtheria was ever found to occur. How do we know in practice whether we are dealing with *Corynebacterium diphtheriæ* or some other bacterium? The organism is recognizable by the fact that it grows very readily on a particular mixture — Loeffler's medium — giving white or cream-colored colonies with a recognizable habit of growth. The microscope shows the bacteria as slightly club-shaped rods about 1/5000 to 1/10,000 of an inch in length, arranged in V- or L-shaped groupings. If cultured in a medium containing cane-sugar, it will produce acid, but it does not attack glucose or malt-sugar. Finally, if a dose of a culture is injected into a guinea-pig it will die in one to four days and a post-mortem examination will show certain recognizable changes. The results of these experiments can give a strong presumption that we are dealing with the diphtheria bacillus, but not complete certainty; for there are types of bacteria resembling *Corynebacterium diphtheriæ* in almost every respect except its power of producing the disease of diphtheria. A final test to clinch the matter is to take two guinea-pigs and protect one by injection of diphtheria antitoxin, then inject both with the suspected bacteria; if these are the true diphtheria bacillus the protected guinea-pig will survive and the other will die.

Suppose then that this organism *Corynebacterium diphtheriæ* lodges in the throat of someone who is susceptible to it — that is to say, whose tissues are unable to destroy it. It grows and spreads over the throat forming a compact mass of 'false membrane,' but it does not invade other parts of the body. But, as it grows, it gives out an exceedingly deadly poison, which is absorbed through the lining membrane of the throat and circulates with the blood through every organ of the body. It is this poison which causes the serious general illness which the diphtheria patient experiences. Another bacterium which always remains localized in a single part is that which causes tetanus. The bacteria remain in the infected wound while the toxins they produce travel up the nerve sheaths and cause the usually fatal convulsions. There are, however, other parasites which do not remain localized. Thus the parasites of malaria and of plague generally circulate in the bloodstream throughout the body. Some bacteria may either be localized or may invade the whole body: thus the *streptococcus pyogenes* may remain localized in a septic wound, causing mild illness; or, more rarely, may spread through the whole body causing the grave condition of septicæmia or blood-poisoning.

We have hitherto given the agents of disease the general title of 'parasites' or 'germs.' There are, in fact, a large number of very different creatures which may use our body as their host, and thereby cause disease. Large, well-organized parasites such as tape-worms, liver-flukes, hookworms head the list, but we shall have most to say concerning the microscopic or ultramicroscopic organisms which Pasteur or Lister would have classed as 'germs'—a convenient term which is now rather out of fashion. These fall into three chief classes; (1) animal parasites (protozoa); (2) vegetable parasites (bacteria and fungi); (3) filter-passing viruses.

The protozoa are exceedingly minute animals consisting of a single cell with a definite nucleus and sometimes more than one of these. They have some means of locomotion, usually one or more fine whip-lashes (flagella) by the aid of which they can swim through a liquid, and some sort of structures analogous to the muscle of higher animals by which they can move. Some are quite highly organized while others seem to be not much more than a mass of protoplasm, but all are probably much more complex organisms than bacteria. They multiply, as a rule, simply by dividing in two, but in many of them there is also something analogous to sexual reproduction. These parasitic protozoa are for the most part exceedingly small: an average length for a trypanosome might be 1/2000 of an inch. One could put about 1500 of them on one of the full-stops on this page. It must not be thought that protozoa are generally parasitic or producers of disease: the soil swarms with independent free-living forms, as also does water, both salt and fresh. Parasitic protozoa are, in fact, only a small section of an enormous class.

The protozoa are not responsible for many of the diseases with which we are familiar in our country, but they cause an appalling mortality in the tropical countries, both among men and among animals. The chief diseases which they cause in man are amœbic dysentery, malaria, sleeping-sickness, leishmaniasis (kala-azar), and if, as is usual, we class the spirochæte as protozoa, relapsing fever and syphilis. In animals they cause the Nagana cattle plague of Africa, surra pest in India, Texas fever of cattle, malignant jaundice of dogs, African coastal fever — all sources of enormous economic loss, but rather unfamiliar to dwellers in temperate climates.

The parasitic protozoa do not often pass directly from one animal to another, probably because they cannot survive for an appreciable time outside the favorable conditions of an animal host. Their usual mode of transmission is by the agency of insects which become infected by sucking blood—and with it parasites—from an infected animal; when the insect bites a second animal, it injects into it some of the parasites, so passing on the infection. This is probably the reason why they are rare in temperate climates in which through a considerable season of the year flying insects are rare.

The chief diseases of temperate climates are caused by a very different class of organism, namely, bacteria. The terms bacterium, germ, bacillus, microbe, etc., are often used as if interchangeable. *Germ* and *microbe* are words belonging to the era before we knew the natural history of these organisms, but may conveniently be used to denote any unspecified microscopic parasite. *Bacterium* is the correct term for the whole class which we are now discussing; the word *bacillus* covers a certain class of bacteria, though it is often loosely used to cover the whole class. By no means all bacteria are parasites, and indeed, since the fertility of the soil is dependent on the activity of bacteria, plant life, and therefore animal life, could not continue without them.

Bacteria are considered to be plants rather than animals, though they bear little resemblance to the common conception either of an animal or a plant. They are exceedingly small — much smaller than most protozoa — and the full-stop on which one could place 1500 average parasitic protozoa would need 250,000 average-sized bacteria to cover it. They consist, like protozoa, of a single cell, but, unlike them, they are covered with a cell-wall which seems to act as a sort of protective capsule. They have no definite nuclei but seem to contain particles of nuclear substances. Some of them can move by means of flagella, but others remain immobile. Little if any organization can be detected in their bodies, but this is not to say that such organization does not exist. Generally speaking, they are rod shaped — when they are known as *bacilli,* or spehrical — when they are known as *cocci.* Actually the appearance of most species of bacteria is extremely variable and we classify them rather by their habits and effects than by their outward appearance. They have no sex and multiply simply by dividing in two. When food is plentiful and all conditions are favorable, they may divide every twenty or thirty minutes. A simple calculation shows that one bacterium could in twelve hours rise to a thousand million descendants — a fact which helps to explain the speed with which a few bacteria introduced into the blood-stream may invade the whole body. In practice this rate of progress is usually limited by lack of foodstuffs and the deleterious effect of the bacterium's own waste products. Some bacteria can form spores, which are very minute bodies highly resistant to heat, cold, and drought; these under favorable conditions germinate once more into active bacteria.

Bacteria cause a great many of our most common and fatal diseases. There follows a list of the commonest parasitic bacteria and the diseases they cause.

Some Disease Bacteria

Streptococus pyogenes (β-hæmolytic streptococcus). Under this title are grouped at least thirty different strains of bacteria differing slightly in their habits. Usual cause of septic wounds, cellulitis, blood-poisoning, erysipelas, puerperal fever, scarlet fever, etc.

Streptococcus pneumoniæ (pneumonococcus). At least thirty-four strains. Usual cause of pneumonia. Occasionally infects organs other than lung.

Staphylococcus aureus. Common inhabitant of skin. Usual cause of boils, frequent in septic wounds.

Neisseria gonorrhœa (gonococcus). Gonorrhœa. Can also infect eyes or joints.

Neisseria meningitis (meningococcus). Cerebrospinal meningitis.

Corynebacterium diphtheriæ. Diphtheria.

Mycobacterium tuberculosis. Tuberculosis.

Vibrio choleræ. Cholera.

Pasteurella pestis. Plague.

Clostridium welchii. One of the bacteria causing gasgangrene.

Clostridium tetani. Lock-jaw.

Bacillus coli. Inhabitant of large intestine. Sometimes infects other organs.

Bacillus anthracis. Anthrax (Woolsorters' disease).

These bacteria are so small and so transparent that it is usually impossible to find them when a specimen of untreated blood or tissue is examined with the microscope, and little could be done until the techniques of rendering them visible and of cultivating them had been perfected. So from about 1880 a new department of science —bacteriology—had to be evolved. The first need was to be able to see the bacteria. This was rendered possible by advances in two other sciences. First of these was the perfection of the microscope by the devising of more elaborate lenses. Higher magnification was not needed, but greater power of resolution — sharper and brighter images in which finer details could be perceived. The second was the production of the basic aniline dyes which were first introduced between 1875 and 1880.

The procedure required to render bacteria visible is to stain material containing them with a solution of a dye, and then to remove the dye from the material as far as possible by means of alcohol, acids, etc. The desired result is that the bacteria should be strongly colored in such a way as to distinguish them from the surrounding tissues: the skill of the bacteriologist is in devising effective methods of staining, this is often no easy task, and scores of methods have been worked out to cover the more difficult cases.

Bacteria are very much alike and cannot always be identified with the microscope. In order to identify them more certainly, and in order to study them in detail, they must be cultivated. Here again the utmost skill is needed. Many bacteria have remained unculturable for years, until some suitable medium has been devised. Difficulties are often caused by the existence of different strains of a bacillus. Thus the pneumococcus is readily recognized, but more exact research shows that there are some thirty-four strains or races of it, which, though they produce similar effects on the body, are not identical, for a serum made from one will not protect against the others. More virulent and less virulent types of the same bacterium exist, and the more virulent bacteria may breed less virulent descendants if cultured under unfavorable circumstances.

In order to know if a bacterium one has cultured is identical with one which has been previously described, it is obviously desirable to compare the two. For this purpose the Lister Institute at Elstree, England, maintains the National Collection of Type Cultures, a zoo of living bacteria — thousands of strains being kept alive, so that any bacteriologist can at any time have access to any type of living bacterium. The standard method, so to speak, of separating a particular kind of bacterium from a fluid which is likely to contain many different kinds is to add a little of the material to be examined to a larger quantity of some sort of jelly in which most bacteria readily grow. By warming the jelly it is liquefied and the bacteria become distributed through the whole of the liquid. The jelly is then poured out into shallow glass dishes. These are incubated. Each separate bacterium multiplies into a little colony of its own single species which can be seen and examined separately, and when the colony of the required bacterium has been found it can be transferred into some suitable culture medium and cultivated to any desired extent. We recognize our bacterium not only by its appearance under the microscope and the stains it takes, but also by its behavior. Some bacteria produce acids when they grow, some produce gas bubbles, some will curdle milk and some will not. Such tests may identify the bacterium: if they do not it is usually possible to inoculate an animal with the culture and examine the symptoms it produces.

But protozoa and bacteria do not exhaust the list of microscopic parasites which affect us. If a liquid containing disease bacteria is filtered through unglazed porcelain the bacteria are too large to penetrate its pores and are held back. The filtered liquid contains no particles visible even by the aid of the best microscope, and it will not communicate the disease to an animal. Now there are a large number of diseases which resemble bacterial diseases in the way they are caught, in their prevalence as epidemics, and indeed in every respect — except that no bacteria can be found. If a body fluid—serum, saliva, etc. — from an animal infected with one of these diseases be filtered through unglazed porcelain it passes through, but remains capable of transmitting the infection to other animals. The microscope shows nothing, but refined physical methods show that the filtered liquid contains particles from a quarter to perhaps a hundredth of the diameter of a bacterium. These have been termed virus-particles and they are the causative agent in many very common diseases of men, other animals, and even plants. Among the diseases of men due to filter-passing viruses, are small-pox, infantile paralysis, typhus fever, common colds, and probably measles, mumps, and influenza; among virus diseases of animals are foot-and-mouth disease, bovine pleuro-pneumonia, swine-fever, canine distemper, and many others.

Why should we regard these virus-particles as living parasites? Partly from analogy with bacteria — for there is no certain dividing line between small bacteria and large virus-particles; but more certainly because they assimilate and reproduce. If a tiny speck of foot-and-mouth disease virus is inoculated into a cow an enormous quantity of it can be recovered from the sick animal, and this power to assimilate foreign matter and reproduce its kind is the chief characteristic of a living thing. The virus particles cannot as a rule be cultivated except in living media, such as an animal's body, a tissue culture, or, very advantageously, a developing hen's egg. The virus particle would seem to have little or no power of breaking down chemical compounds — of digestion, in fact — but has to rely on the ready-made food-material in the cell itself.

The practical use of our knowledge about parasitic protozoa, bacteria, and viruses is to enable us to prevent or cure the diseases they cause. Speaking very generally it may be said that, other things being equal, we have most control over the most highly organized parasites. Neglecting the special difficulties created by tropical conditions, primitive habits, and the like, it may be said that we know how to prevent and how to cure most of the diseases caused by protozoa; that we know how to prevent most bacterial diseases and how to cure some of them; while with a very few exceptions we are not generally able to do much to prevent the spread of virus diseases nor do we know any specific methods of aiding the body in its efforts to overcome them.

The germ-theory of disease was established in the early 'eighties, but it did very little towards teaching us how to cure germ-diseases until this century was under way. But it did teach us to prevent them. We still have no very effective means of curing typhoid fever, tuberculosis, smallpox, scarlet fever, measles, whooping cough, but there died in England from these causes in

each of the years 1876-1880, 7474 peoples per million living: in the years 1931-1935, but 1740! One
cannot, of course, attribute the whole drop in
mortality to the germ-theory and its teaching —
yet this was undoubtedly the chief cause of the
decrease.

The germ-theory of disease taught us a great
many things which seem to-day to be wholly obvious, but which were by no means so in 1870. It
taught us that to prevent disease we must keep dis-
ease-organisms out of the body. It showed that
the routes by which they entered the body were

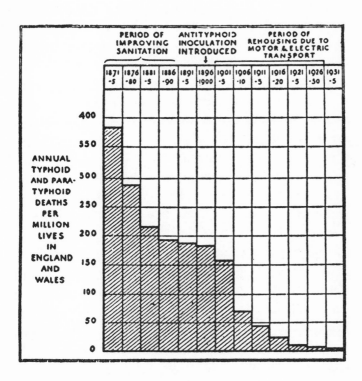

with air, water, food, dirty wounds, and insect-
bites: it also showed that some bacteria (e.g. the
pneumococcus and streptococcus) were quite
common inhabitants of our bodies, and that they
caused trouble only when they multiplied in some
part of the body which was not their normal habitat.   The germ-theory thus made us aware of the
need for national hygiene, and sixty years of education, newspaper publicity, and advertisement have
begun to make hygiene a national habit.

As we mentioned on page 17, the nineteenth
century believed that diseases were carried by a
bad smell, and so, when it felt itself hygienically
inclined, it opened the windows.   There was,
moreover, an early period in the germ-theory of
disease, when as a result of Pasteur's and Lister's
work, the air was looked on as the chief means of
transmitting disease-germs.   Our point of view has
altered somewhat; we know now that some germs
are commonly carried by the air and that others
are rarely if ever transmitted in this way.   If you
sneeze, cough, or even speak vigorously before a
sheet of glass tiny droplets of saliva and mucus
will settle upon it.   These are charged with many
bacteria or virus particles which were inhabitants
of the mouth of the speaker.   In a well-ventilated
place such droplets will be quickly carried up
the chimney or out of the window; in a dry place
they will quickly evaporate — which is enough to
kill a good many bacteria.   But if the air is still,
and if it is humid, the droplets will stand a good
chance of being inhaled by other people; and if

their mouths and noses are good culture-media
they will probably catch the disease. It is believed that the common cold, influenza, cerebrospinal meningitis, and most of the common epidemic diseases of childhood are thus acquired. It
is not easy to prevent the transmission of diseases
in this way as long as we inhabit overcrowded
houses, pack into railroad coaches, and generally
crowd together in unventilated places. Some of
these diseases, such as influenza, are apparently so
infectious that whether precautions are taken or
not, the susceptible are very likely to catch them,
while others such as infantaile paralysis infect only
a very small proportion of contacts. Generally
speaking, it is true to say that living and effective
bacteria of disease are very rarely carried through
the air for more than a few feet.

Some bacteria are conveyed into the body by
way of water or food taken into the alimentary
system. Water is to-day subjected to the most vigorous inspection. It is usually drawn from deep
wells into which it has filtered through a vast
sponge of chalk, or from lakes in uninhabited
moorland; if it has to be taken from a suspect
source, such as the Thames, it is filtered and often
disinfected by means of chlorine. Dirty water, as
such, is not particularly harmful; the danger is in
water polluted to however small an extent with
human excreta. Sufferers from typhoid and paratyphoid fevers, from dysentery, or from Asiatic
cholera discharge in their excreta vast numbers of
the bacteria of these diseases. If these by devious

routes enter a source of drinking-water, they may infect anyone who drinks it. In London, until the 'seventies, we used to discharge our sewage into the Thames, and in the 'forties some of the water companies supplied practically untouched Thames water to the houses of Londoners. The result was that in the 'forties one Londoner in forty-one died of typhoid; to-day one in three thousand does so. Cholera carried off 13,000 people in 1849 alone: it is now unknown in England, but in India it carried off over a million people in 1918-1919. The means of prevention of these two diseases is perfectly understood; the difficulty of their prevention lies in the education of people not to drink filth, and much more in persuading someone to pay for clean water supplies and hygienic sewage-disposal.

Solid food is not often a source of infection, and any food that is properly cooked becomes sterilized. The most dangerous forms of food are shell-fish which have grown in water polluted with sewage. It is estimated that in France during the fifteen years after the war of 1914-1918 more than 100,000 cases of typhoid fever were caused by eating shell-fish and that they resulted in 25,000 deaths.

The most dangerous — as well as perhaps the best — of all foods is milk. Milk as it comes from the cow is fairly free from bacteria, provided that the cow is not suffering from disease. Where precautions are not taken to see that the cows are healthy, streptococci and tubercle bacilli may be present in the new milk at the rate of hundreds in every drop.   Milk is an ideal culture medium for bacteria, and most of those which enter it will live and grow.   Unsterilized pails, cans, coolers, and so forth may contribute bacteria, mostly the harmless types which cause milk to become sour. The milker's hands contribute other bacteria. These may be harmless and, perhaps, usually are so.   But a small proportion of the population are *carriers* of disease bacteria, by which we mean that they harbor the bacteria in their intestines, bladders, or throats, without suffering from the disease itself.   It may happen, then, that a milker may be a source of diphtheria, scarlet fever, typhoid, or dysentery germs, and such a person is a serious threat to the community.

Milking and milk-handling really demands — and sometimes gets — a sort of surgical technique. But human institutions are imperfect, so where milk from many sources is mixed — as is common in the supply of great towns — it is best that milk should be pasteurized.   The milk is heated to 145° - 150° F. and held at that temperature for half an hour, then quickly cooled to 55° F. or less.   This kills all bacteria which can cause disease and does not affect the flavor of the milk. There is no objection to the process except the almost fatal one that it costs a little money.

Dirt — in the sense of what is seen on dirty hands — is not often a source of infectious disease.   It does, however, harbor a great many bacteria — especially of the hardier sorts. Dirt of this kind in a wound is likely to make it become septic, but only in a very small proportion of cases do superficial dirty cuts lead to serious trouble. Deep wounds such as are caused by a nail or a needle running into the flesh are to be treated with much more respect. The really dangerous dirt is well-manured earth or horse-dung (for those often contain the deadly tetanus bacillus), and decomposing animal matter such as is contained in sewage, which commonly contains the streptococci which may give rise to blood-poisoning.

The bites of insects are a very important means of distributing bacteria. In our country, where biting flies are few and for many months of the year are not to be found, and where lice, fleas, bugs, and ticks are harbored only by a small section of the population, insect-borne disease is not serious; but in tropical climates and among primitive people who are commonly verminous these diseases reach gigantic proportions. Generally speaking, the infection is spread by the insect's sucking blood from a diseased person and so becoming infected with the bacteria, which it injects into the next person whom it bites; but in some cases the disease is carried by insects which do not bite but which merely carry bacteria on their feet or mouth parts. Thus in this country during the hot months the disease of summer diarrhœa is fatal to a great number of infants. It appears that it is spread chiefly by flies settling first on the excreta of infected children and then on the food of others. The disease but rarely attacks breast-fed infants, and it is most prevalent in the dirtiest homes and at the times of year when flies most prevail. Typhoid fever and dysentery are some-times carried by flies in this same manner, but only, it would seem, where flies are very prevalent and where there is no sanitary system, e.g. in primitive Eastern cities, amongst armies in hot countries, etc.

Mosquitoes are carriers of malaria, which is responsible for several million deaths every year, and o1 the far less prevalent but much more deadly yellow fever. They also carry an unpleasant tropical fever known as dengue. The extermina-tion of mosquitoes would abolish these diseases, but this is impossible to accomplish except in civil-ized communities. Town districts can be cleared of mosquitoes by making it impossible for their larvæ — the familiar water-butt wrigglers — to breed. By draining swamps, covering ponds with films of oil or the arsenical poison Paris Green, their breeding grounds can be abolished, and the disease disappears with the mosquito. But it is impossible to clear miles of swampy jungle of pools — and a mere quart of water in the hollow of a dead tree will breed its dozens of these insects. The tsetse fly, which carries sleeping-sickness and the cattle plague which makes a good part of Africa inaccessible to horses and cows, is harder to deal with than the mosquito, and there seems at present not much hope of exterminating it ex-

cept in very limited areas. Finally the human parasites — fleas and lice — can carry deadly diseases. The flea and the rat together carry plague.
Certain rodents, notably the tarbagans of Mon-
golia, suffer from epidemics of plague: they are
the reservoirs of the bacterium *Pasteurella pestis*.
They infect the fleas with which they are infested.
These move from the dying animals to other
rodents, notably rats. Rats travel with ships and
trains or migrate, as rats will, from village to village. Populations whose houses are infested with
rats and with fleas become bitten by the fleas. The
fore-stomach of the plague-infected flea becomes
blocked with plague bacteria and it is forced to
regurgitate into the bite some of the blood it has
sucked — and with it the plague bacteria. The
persons bitten contract plague and from two-
thirds to nine-tenths die of it. The means of
prevention are obvious — not to be infested with
fleas and rats. As populations adopt civilized
habits, plague disappears, but in India it kills, on
the average, half a million people every year. It is
possible to wonder whether, if a very small part
of the money we spend on making war, preparing
for war, and paying for past wars, could be spent
on the extermination of the Asian rodents which
are the originators of plague, this vast wastage of
life could not be wholly abolished.

Typhus fever is carried from man to man by the
louse. The louse goes out when laundries and
baths come in, and so typhus has disappeared
from the Western world. But when a louse-

infested population in a low health is crowded together, typhus is likely to sweep through it. The armies of the Crimea, the Serbian populations in the war of 1914-1918, were subject to great epidemics. Despite the high lousiness of the armies on the Western Front in 1914-1918, typhus did not prevail. In its stead there appeared another louse-born disease — trench fever — somewhat resembling typhus but far less deadly.

Once the mode of transport of bacteria is known, prevention usually becomes possible. But there is more than one kind of possibility. Before a preventive method can be successful it must be scientifically possible, humanly possible, and economically possible. It is scientifically possible to abolish typhoid, cholera, malaria, plague and typhus. In England, most European countries, and the U.S.A., it is also humanly possible: for we can persuade or compel most of the population to behave in a moderately hygienic fashion and we have educated them to the stage of preferring not to harbor vermin. In these countries it is also economically possible, for they can afford, and are willing to carry out, the necessary hygienic work, to provide clean water, to dispose of sewage, to inspect food and milk, isolate infectious persons, and so forth. In more primitive countries it is not humanly or economically possible to control these diseases. It is often impossible to persuade the inhabitants that rats, fleas, and lice, are objectionable house-mates, that the nearest pool is not necessarily the best water, and that the nearest place is not necessarily the best dump for their sewage and household waste. Such communities can only be 'cleaned up' against their will — or at least without their co-operation. Moreover, such communities are poor. They cannot afford great schemes of sewerage, water-supply, swamp-drainage, mosquito-control, and so forth, unless richer communities are willing and able to pay for them.

So it must be realized that preventive medicine has human limitations as well as scientific ones. Where it has been given its fullest scope it has nearly abolished typhoid, cholera, plague, malaria, and typhus, and, by isolation of patients, has much diminished the incidence of common infectious diseases, such as measles, whooping-cough, scarlet fever, and the like. Yet even at its most efficient, preventive medicine can only diminish the prevalence of these common epidemics, and there is, moreover, a class of bacterial diseases for which it can do almost nothing. These are the diseases caused by bacteria which are normal inhabitants of the human body. Streptococci — which are responsible for most septic wounds and blood poisoning and many other diseases — are common in decomposing organic matter and, indeed, in all sorts of dust and dirt. Our noses and throats always contain streptococci; these may be of fairly harmless type, but one person in about fifteen harbors virulent ones as well. The human nose and throat usually also contain living pneumococci, staphylococci, and bacteria resembling but not, as a rule, identical with those which cause dipththeria. The human skin always contains staphylococci — the organisms which cause boils and pimples. Every human large intestine contains more bacteria at a time than there are people in the world. These are harmless — it is generally thought — as long as they stay there, but they can cause trouble if they gain access to other organs. Preventive medicine can do very little to prevent people becoming generally infected from germs they carry about with them, though it can do a good deal to prevent one person's germs from travelling to another. Thus it can do little, if anything, to prevent pneumonia, or tonsillitis, but it can do a great deal by surgical precautions to prevent these throat-dwelling bacteria from reaching places where they would cause havoc, such as clean wounds or the genital tract of women in childbirth.

It should be clear, then, that although prevention may be preferable to cure, cure is going to remain necessary for the diseases which science cannot prevent, and also for those which can prevent only by methods which society will not adopt or cannot afford. It must be remembered, too, that cure and prevention tend to the same result for, at least in some cases, cure of the sick is a means of preventing the spread of the disease to the healthy. If, for example, a whole community can be simultaneously cured of malaria and kept free from it for a mosquito's short life-time, there will be no malaria parasites left in the district to infect the mosquitoes. It is thus theoretically possible for such disease parasites as can only live in human beings to be completely wiped out of a community. Thus if there were a system of compulsory medical examination and treatment for all, the venereal diseases could be completely wiped out of a community, for their parasites only exist in man and rarely, if ever, inhabit people who do not suffer from the disease. Such a system we should feel to be too expensive and a violation of personal freedom; as a community we prefer venereal disease to compulsory examination, and quite possibly we are right.

Some parasites, then, we might stamp out, but others, it would seem, must continue to infect us and cause illness which we must fight as best we may. There are two main weapons we can use: first, those based on nature's own mode of warfare — namely, antitoxins, vaccines, sera, inoculation and the like — secondly, synthetic drugs which kill bacteria within the tissues. The two methods rarely overlap, for, generally speaking, the first is conspicuously successful where the second fails, and vice versa.

CHAPTER II

THE BODY'S DEFENSES

Exclusion of bacteria — Macrophages — Immunology — Inoculation and Vaccination — Antitoxins — Serum-therapy.

THE parts of the body which do not come into direct contact with matter from the outer world are practically free from bacteria. The nose and throat are continually in contact with air, and the alimentary canal with food; these swarm with bacteria. But even in these sites the bacterial flora is limited. There are a dozen or so types of bacteria which are common in the mouth and cannot be removed from it; yet if a new species is introduced it commonly fails to keep its footing there and is washed away and swallowed. In the same way only a few species of bacteria can flourish in the human intestine, and most species either fail to get there, being destroyed by the acid of the stomach, or once there, dwindle away and disappear. But what we usually describe as the 'internal organs' of a healthy body are free from bacteria. And they are not merely free from them as a sealed tin of lobster is free. Bacteria are not merely excluded from the tissues of the body; but when they gain entrance, as organisms so nearly ubiquitous occasionally must, they are systematically attacked and destroyed. A living man whose organs have been practically free from bacteria for half a century is killed on a hot summer's day by a car accident: within forty-eight hours the organs of the corpse will be swarming with bacteria — the progenitors of which were all in his intestines, skin, throat, etc., while he was alive, but were continually removed and destroyed as and when they penetrated his living tissues. Clearly the living body is constantly at watch and ward to destroy bacteria, and no living organism — plant or animal — could exist without some means of destroying them. It is natural to expect that a very elaborate defense should have been evolved to meet a need so primitive and so essential.

The body has several lines of defense. In the first place the whole of its tissues is protected from the outside world by various kinds of membrane or skin. Our exterior skin is normally impermeable to bacteria. Staphylocci always live on its surface, but normally cannot penetrate it, though sometimes they grow down into a sweat-gland and cause a pimple, or into a hair-follicle and cause a boil, so calling the body's second line of defense into action. Most other bacteria cannot even live for long on clean skin which has definite germicidal powers. The interiors of our mouths, stomachs, and intestines are lined with a more delicate skin. This is a little more readily infected, but has further defenses against infection. The mouth is continually washed with saliva, causing most unusual bacteria to be swallowed. The stomach's contents are so acid that hardly any bacteria pass out of it alive. The intestines, however. swarm with bacteria — nearly half of our fæces, indeed, consists of the bodies of bacteria — but these cannot penetrate the intestinal wall. The air-passages of the nose and throat naturally abound with bacteria, for one of their functions is to entrap the solid particles from the air we breathe against their moist surface. This process renders the air which enters the lungs moderately sterile, and nearly all the remaining bacteria deposit on the walls of the larger air-tubes of the lungs — the bronchi — and become entangled in mucus. Very fine hair-like processes — cilia — which project into the air-way waft the mucus and bacteria up the windpipe to the mouth, from which they are harmlessly swallowed and destroyed in the stomach. There is probably another mechanism of removal via the lymphatic vessels. This elaborate system of purifying the air keeps the delicate membrane between the air and blood in the lungs from attack.

Thus the body has various mechanisms for keeping out bacterial invaders but these are not entirely efficient as we see by the fact that we do catch illnesses of many kinds. So the body requires and possesses further lines of defense against such bacteria as may penetrate the skin or mucous membrane. Let us suppose that a few

hundred thousand bacteria have in some way penetrated the outer defenses and entered the blood-
stream.   The blood circulates so rapidly that within
a minute or two they will have travelled round
the whole circulation.   Throughout the body there
are countless cells, which we call *macrophages;*
these are specialized to do one particular job —
picking up and engulfing any foreign particles.
Most of these are found in the 'reticulo-endo-
thelial system,' that is to say, lining the tiny blood-
vessels of the liver, bone-marrow, and other organs; but some wander about the body freely or
even circulate in the blood.   The blood also contains certain types of white cells or leucocytes
which have much the same function as the macrophages.   These macrophages pick up most of or
all of the bacteria and generally destroy them,
and they can usually overcome any small infection.   If the bacteria are of a fairly mild type this
is almost certain to be their fate.   But if the
bacteria are virulent and actively multiplying they
may survive in the sites where they have been
captured and even multiply there, so forming
centres of infection — strong-posts as it were —
in which they hold out for some time.   If they are
very virulent they may multiply to such an extent
as to enter the blood-stream again and so spread
through the whole body.   When this has occurred
the body is thrown on its third line of defense —
the production of substances which kill the bacteria
and destroy the toxins they have produced.
We have considered the case where the bac-

teria have entered the blood-stream. But there are many cases where they do not do so. Thus when staphylococci infect a hair follicle and produce a boil there is no invasion of the blood-stream, but a purely local quarrel. The blood-vessels round the hair follicle become dilated. Near the centre the blood-flow is retarded or even ceases. Fluid escapes through the walls of the blood-vessels and large numbers of macrophages and leucocytes migrate to the infected centre. The bacteria are then poisoned by the special substances which the body makes and their remains and the dead and damaged tissue may be cleared up by the macrophages. But if this debris is at all considerable in quantity, it forms the liquid we call pus. This consists of dead and living leucocytes and bacteria which have been digested to a fluid, which usually escapes by bursting through the skin.

So whether in a local disease or a general one, the body has two quite different mechanisms, the engulfing of bacteria by macrophages and the destruction of them and their poisons by chemical substances which it has the power to make; and in most diseases the last is the decisive factor. If the body can produce these chemical antidotes at such a rate that they kill the bacteria quicker than they can multiply, the bacteria die out and the body wins. If these antidotes are not quite so effective they may clear the bacteria from the general circulation but fail to expel them from certain strongholds. This produces a chronic illness which may be hardly noticeable or may be serious. Most of us are or have at some time been on such terms of drawn-out siege-warfare with streptococci in our tonsils and tubercle bacilli in our lymphatic glands or lungs. Lastly the bacterium may multiply more rapidly than the antidotes can destroy it and may invade the body to such an extent that its poisons cause death.

A whole department of science, known as Immunology, deals with the manner in which the body prepares and employs these chemical weapons. Since we shall be talking about the poisons the bacteria produce and also the poisons by which the body destroys the bacteria, it will be best if we adopt the scientific terminology. The bacterial poisons, and, generally, anything which, when introduced into the tissues causes them to produce a substance which will react with it, and, as a rule, render it harmless, is called an *antigen,* and the new substance produced by the body is called an *antibody*. Generally each antigen causes the formation of a special antibody which will react with it and with it alone. Thus diphtheria toxin (p. 25) injected into a horse stimulates it to produce diphtheria antitoxin. This will combine with and destroy diphtheria toxin, but will have no effect on any other toxin, e.g. that of tetanus.

The body has, then, a mechanism by which it can produce an antidote to any poison of a certain class. Not, mark you, to any poison whatever, for the body cannot produce an antibody to simple chemical substances as arsenic or strychnine. It can produce antibodies only to certain proteins (probably those derived from the amino-acid tyrosine) and to certain complicated carbo-hydrates such as the gums. In these classes are included bacteria and their poisonous products.

The grand principle by which the body deals with foreign invasion may then be summed up as:

(1)   The invading material contains one or more *antigens* and provokes the tissues to form one or more *antibodies*.

(2)   The antigens and antibodies combine to-gether and form some harmless, inert substance.

With a non-living poison, such as snake-venom or diphtheria toxin, this process is all that occurs. If, however, the body is invaded by living bac-teria the process is a little more complicated. Bac-teria contain a number of chemical substances which act as antigens and provoke the body to form antibodies which combine with parts of the bacteria. The first of these are agglutinins. They modify the surface of the bacteria and make them 'stick' so that they clot into clumps which macro-phages and leucocytes find it easy to 'swallow' and remove. The second are bacteriolysins which profoundly modify the bacteria with the aid of a mysterious substance called *complement* which is found in the serum of the blood. So to destroy our bacteria:

(1)   Tissues produce antibodies of two types — agglutinins and bacteriolysins.

(2)   Agglutinin and normal bacteria/'sticky' bacteria.

(3)   Sticky bacteria clump together and are removed by macrophages.

At the same time:

(4)   Bacteriolysins sensitize the bacteria to the poisonous action of complement in the serum.

(5)   Complement kills the bacteria.

Each species of bacterium requires a different agglutinin and bacteriolysin, but the same complement is destructive to all.

At first sight is seems almost miraculous that the body should be able to make a separate remedy for any of the scores of thousands of possible protein poisons. This power may be a marvel but it is clearly also a necessity, for otherwise if a bacterium evolved a new poison, as almost certainly sometimes occurs, the body would have no defense for it and the race would be extirpated. It is pretty certain that there is some sort of mechanism by which each poison automatically evokes its appropriate remedy. Many theories have been put forward to explain this. Ehrlich supposed that the bacterial poison or in, general terms, each antigen *combined* with some special part of the tissue-molecule, and so put it out of action. The formation of antibody was, he supposed, the production by the cell of a great number of free 'spare-parts' of this special kind. These entered the blood-stream and combined with the antigen before it could reach the fixed 'part' in the tissue cell. The difficulty which has led to the rejection of this famous theory is that the tissues seem to be able to make an unlimited number of different antibodies, whereas they cannot have an unlimited number of 'parts.' According to another theory the body modifies each antigen and makes it into an antibody. This would account for there being a separate antibody for every antigen, but the fatal objection seems to be that the quantity of antibody produced much exceeds that of the antigen introduced! Generally speaking, we must be content to accept the fact that the body performs the feat, almost incredible to the chemist, of synthesizing antibodies capable of rendering harmless any of some thousands — perhaps millions — of antigens.

The body then has strong weapons against bacteria in the form of macrophages and antibodies. The defect of the latter defense is that it does not begin to operate until the bacterium or poison enters the system. There is then a race between the multiplication of the bacteria or their production of poisons, and the manufacture of antibodies. The body is like a very powerful nation with a very small standing army. If it has time to muster its forces it is likely to win, but it may be conquered by a *blitzkrieg*. Even if the bacteria lose the battle, they commonly get a run for their money and cause grave illness during the period while the body is manufacturing its antibodies. Thus in many diseases we have these stages:

(1) Infection with a few bacteria.
(2) Unsuccessful attempt to sweep up and destroy these (p. 52).

During this time nothing may be noticed, but when the bacteria become plentiful, there occur:

(4)   Illness due to toxins produced by bacteria.

(5)   Production of antibodies by tissues.

Followed by either:

(6)   Death of bacteria and destruction of toxins, and recovery of patient.

or

(7)   Death of patient poisoned by bacterial toxins.

The issue of death or recovery then depends on the result of the race between multiplication of bacteria and production of antibodies. The bacteria are much less likely to win the race if the body has before their arrival a ready-made stock of appropriate antibodies or if, during the race, we can add artificially to its store.

For very many years we have known that there are diseases from which a patient rarely suffers twice; thus, for example, an attack of small-pox makes a person *immune* to further attacks. The immunity is in most cases not permanent, but as a rule there is a period, short or long, after the recovery from a disease in which it is not contracted again. We explain this by supposing that during the disease the body produces more antibodies than it needs to destroy the bacteria and toxins, and that these antibodies remain in the system for a certain time and destroy any bacteria of the same kind the moment they enter the system and before they have time to multiply. Most adults are thus protected against measles, mumps, whooping-cough, and such childish ailments as they have passed through. But they also become protected against others which they have not had. It is a common practice to test the skin with diphtheria toxin to see whether the person tested is susceptible to the disease. If he is so, the skin becomes inflamed: if he is not, it is unaffected. It is found that most young children are susceptible but that only a few adults are so. The reason is supposed to be that we all get small doses of diphtheria germs from time to time and cope with them without even becoming ill. By so doing we build up a stock of antibodies and become immune. The same is true of tuberculosis. Probably 97 per cent of us adults would show healed tuberculous lestions if we were carefully dissected. Thus, generally speaking, we all have very mild tuberculosis at some time and develop an immunity. When Europeans take their tuberculosis to communities in which the disease has been unknown, e.g. the inhabitants of some of the Pacific islands — the unprotected population suffers a fearful mortality.

Most of us adults are thus fortified against some of the common ailments, but there are others against which there is little natural immunity on which to depend. In some of these cases, though by no means all, we may protect ourselves by provoking the tissues to produce the necessary antibodies.

This plan was invented long before anybody had thought of disease-germs — let alone antibodies. Smallpox was in past centuries a fatal and disfiguring disease. In our country today it causes a negligible mortality, but in India it still causes some fifty thousand deaths every year. There seems to be a severe and a mild form of the disease. It is not caused by bacteria but by virus-particles. One attack of the disease has long been known to confer complete immunity, and at one time nearly every person suffered from the disease: indeed, it is said that, in the Middle Ages, not to be pock-marked was, *ipso facto,* to be beautiful. In the Near East in the sixteenth and seventeenth centuries, the practice of inoculation grew up. A very mild case of smallpox would be sought, and children would be inoculated with it by rubbing the matter from pustules into cuts, in much the same fashion as we are vaccinated today. The inoculated children developed a mild form of the disease, were not as a rule much inconvenienced or appreciably marked, and were protected for life from the disease. Lady Mary Wortley Montagu, who was the wife of the Ambassador at Constantinople, had her own boy inoculated in 1718 and brought the practice to England. In 1796 Jenner discovered that a disease of cows — vaccinia or cow-pox — could affect man very mildly and that an attack of it gave protection against smallpox. Jenner thought — and it may well be true — that cow-pox is simply a modified form of smallpox, and that vaccination was just a very safe way of inoculation. Vaccination has become almost universal. There are many anti-vaccinationists who argue very plausibly against it, but the following table, reproduced from Topley and Wilson's *Principles of Bacteriology and Immunity* (1936), tells its tale.

RELATION OF SMALLPOX MORBIDITY TO VACCINATION LAWS
IN THE UNITED STATES, 1919-28

Vaccination Laws	No. of States	Population	No. of Cases	Incidence per 100,000
Compulsory Vaccination	10	32,434,954	21,543	6.6
Local Option .	6	17,930,882	91,981	51.3
No Vaccination Laws .	29	59,923,117	393,924	66.7
Compulsory Vaccination prohibited .	4	4,002,888	46,110	115.2

The theory of inoculation is simple. The attack provokes the tissues to form antibodies which remain in the body for years — though probably not indefinitely. Inoculation cannot, however, be very widely applied because of the difficulty of ensuring that the attack of the disease shall be mild. Pasteur managed to obtain and culture a mild anthrax strain which was used to inoculate cattle and must have saved millions of dollars. A more recent attempt has been the B.C.G. treatment of tuberculosis. Calmette introduced the inoculation of infants with living tubercle bacilli of a strain which had lost its virulence as a result of years of growth on a certain medium. The theory, of course, was that the children would produce antibodies, which would protect them against the attacks of true virulent tubercle bacilli. There is a great deal of controversy as to the value of the method, and in 1935 it demonstrated the danger of inoculation in no uncertain fashion. At Luebeck 251 infants were inoculated and 72 of them died in a few month of tuberculosis. Virulent tubercle bacilli had entered the vaccine—probably as a result of someone's error. But a method in which an error can produce such results must remain suspect.

The possible danger of introducing living bacteria into the body led to a new and very successful technique. Dead bacteria, one may suppose, contain the same antigens as living bacteria and so may be expected to provoke the tissues to produce the same antibodies as will kill living bacteria. 'Stone dead hath no fellow,' and a bacterium well and truly killed cannot multiply; so this method is quite safe — and in many cases very effective in conferring protection.

Typhoid fever has, as we have seen, been largely eliminated from communities which drink clean water, eat clean oysters, and have proper sewerage. But armies in the field, and those who have to live in insanitary communities, cannot avoid infection through flies (p. 42) and contaminated water (p. 40). In the Boer War the cases of typhoid were 105 per 1000 men each year: this showed very clearly the need to protect armies in the field against the disease. Almwroth Wright in 1897 devised a method of doing this. The usual method of applying it to-day is as follows: typhoid and paratyphoid bacilli are cultured and then killed by heating the culture to 55-60° C. for 30-60 minutes. A little carbolic acid is added to preserve them. An injection of 1,250,000,000 dead bacteria followed by a further dose of 2,500,000,000 bacteria a week to a fortnight later, is a strong protection against the disease — at least for a few months. In 1915 the incidence of the disease among inoculated soldiers was about one in ten thousand — among those not inoculated, one in a thousand.

There are a good many obstacles to inoculation and vaccination. There are many disease-parasites which we cannot obtain in mild forms suitable for inoculation, and it is never very desirable to introduce living bacteria. So in actual practice, smallpox is prevented by vaccination with cow-pox virus, the B.C.G. inoculation has been used for tubercle, but is not in much favor; but no other form of inoculation is employed. Cattle are inoculated against anthrax and pigs against swine erysipelas: in these cases sera (p. 66) are also used as a partial protection. Vaccination with dead bacteria is effective as a protection against typhoid, cholera, plague, and whooping-cough, but the protection is not absolute. Protection can also be given against diphtheria and scarlet fever by injecting the toxin (not the bacteria) and the antitoxin at the same time. The former provokes the formation of antibodies and the latter prevents poisoning by the toxin. This is a very short list of diseases, and in fact there are but few diseases against which we can be adequately protected.

Where prevention is not possible we must seek for a cure. When a disease is already in progress vaccination is useless, for the body is probably making its antibodies as quickly as it can: and the addition of more antigens may well do more harm than good by using up the antibodies already formed. To aid the body which is already coping with bacteria, we must supply it with ready-made antibodies.

It is impossible to synthesize antibodies in the chemical works as we synthesize aspirin, for antibodies are proteins and we do not know the chemical formula of any protein: nor indeed, if we knew the formulæ, have we any chemical technique which could avail to make them. So if we want antibodies we must get an animal to make them for us.

The usual procedure is to inject the bacteria, dead, living, or both, into an animal — usually a horse. When enormous doses of bacteria have caused the animal's tissues to make enormous quantities of antibodies, it is bled, the blood-serum is separated from the corpuscles, and preserved in sterile condition. If this is injected into the patient the horse's antibodies will be just as effective as his own, provided that the bacterium which is invading his tissues is identical with that which invaded the horse; this proviso is not always easy to fulfil. If the disease is one in which it is not the bacteria but only their toxins that invade the tissues, the toxin is injected into the horse, and the

serum drawn off will contain the antibody to it —
antitoxin, as it is called. The grand success of this
method is the antitoxin treatment of diphtheria.
The mortality figures for this disease are very
convincing. Here is the mortality per million
people living in Great Britain.

Deaths from diphtheria under 15 years
of age per 1,000,000 living.

1886-1890	. .	799
1891-1895	. .	896
1896-1900	. .	893
1901-1905	. .	668
1906-1910	. .	503
1910-1915	. .	444
1916-1920	. .	449
1920-1925	. .	309
1926-1930	. .	301
1931-1935	. .	300

Antitoxin brought into use from
c. 1895.

Immunization by toxin-antitoxin
mixture from c. 1919.

Another triumph was the use of tetanus antitoxin. In September, 1914, one wounded soldier
in a hundred developed the terrible and fatal
disease of tetanus (p. 27). After a few weeks all
wounded men were injected as a routine with the
antitoxin and for the war as a whole only one
wounded man in every eight hundred and fifty
developed the disease. Moreover, the mortality
of those who did acquire it was more than
halved.

A disadvantage of antitoxin treatment is the
short period for which the immunity lasts. Antibodies produced by an animal and injected into
the human body disappear from it after a short
time. If, on the other hand, the body makes its
own antibodies it acquires a much more lasting
immunity. So it is now a common practice to

inject the toxin and enough antitoxin to prevent deleterious effects, or to inject 'toxoid' which is the bacterial toxin treated with some substance, such as formaldehyde, which renders it harmless yet still capable of provoking the formation of antibodies.

Sera containing antibodies designed to kill bacteria have been used in meningitis, pneumonia, anthrax, gas gangrene, bacillary dysentery, and in diseases caused by the staphylococcus (p. 46) and the streptococci (p. 117). In none of these diseases have the effects been spectacular, though on a long series of cases there is a decided lowering of mortality. One of the chief difficulties has been the existence of different strains of bacteria. Thus there are apparently at least thirty-four strains of pneumococci and a serum prepared from one strain gives either partial or no immunity against the others: the same is true of staphylococci and β-hæmolytic streptococci. These sera have undoubtedly proved valuable, but they have without exception shown a large percentage of cases in which no effect has been produced.

There are, moreover, a great number of bacteria and other parasites against which no effective sera can be produced. Many bacteria and virus particles have little or no effect on animals and so cannot cause them to produce antibodies. Thus for mumps, measles, infantile paralysis, gonorrhœa, syhpilis, no sera can be prepared. The sera which are used for inoculation against colds are not against the cold-virus, but against

the other bacteria (streptococci, etc.) which cause
its unpleasant sequels.

Generally speaking, then, it is only in diphtheria that serum treatment is so effective and
certain that nothing better could be desired. For
other diseases sera are either not available or useless or, at best, a means of treatment which frequently fails. A treatment which frequently fails,
is, of course, not to be rejected, especially where,
as in pneumonia or blood-poisoning, there is no
other means of aiding recovery.

The study of immunology has enormous possibilities, for in all probability there is at least a
theoretical possibility of obtaining an antibody
capable of destroying every toxin and bacterium.
The difficulties are very great. The bacteria are
at the limit of visibility: antigens and antibodies
are proteins which we cannot even isolate in a
state of purity: minute and little understood variations in them are of vital significance. Important researches on this subject are in progress. The
work of Landsteiner, Harington, Goebel, and
others, on synthetic antigens is extremely significant and, at any time, may open the way to
further technical mastery. But, at the moment,
the eyes of the world are on another means of
treating parasitic diseases, which in a limited,
but most important field has scored significant
triumphs.

CHAPTER III

THE DEVELOPMENT OF DRUGS

Attempts to kill parasites within the body — Early work on drugs — Organic chemistry — Chemical formulæ — The rise of synthetic drugs—The drug industry—Chemotherapy.

WHILE bacteriologists were conducting their experiments on the prevention and cure of parasitic disease by means of vaccines and sera, the possibility of destroying the parasite, the root and cause of the disease, by other means had not been entirely neglected. Preventive medicine and antiseptic surgery had shown us by the early 'eighties exactly how bacteria could be killed. All of them could be killed by heat. Some were destroyed at quite low temperatures such as 140° F., but others needed prolonged boiling before all trace of life was extinguished. The spores of certain bacteria seemed particularly resistant. It was obviously impossible to heat the human body, for once its temperature reaches 107-110° F. extensive damage and even death may occur. Yet this method has had some applications. A few bacteria and protozoa are very sensitive to heat, and are largely destroyed when the human body is heated to 103-105° F. The organisms which cause gonorrhœa and syphilis are very sensitive to such treatment. Syphilis, in its late nervous manifestations, has been successfully treated by raising the patient's temperature. This can be done by infecting him with malaria — a disease in which periods of high temperature naturally occur — and then curing the malaria with quinine. Other agents besides malaria parasites can be used to provoke the rise of temperature. Gonorrhœa germs have a way of entrenching themselves in some recess of the genito-urinary system. They can usually be dislodged by dosing the patient with sulphonamide drugs (Chapter IX), but in the small proportion of cases where these prove ineffective they can sometimes be destroyed by heat. It is not possible to heat the interior of the body by any of the ordinary ways of applying warmth. The heat must be generated inside the body itself. One way of doing this is by diathermy, that is, subjecting the parts to a powerful high-tension electric current oscillating at such an enormous frequency that it gives no shock and has no effect except that of heating the tissues in its path. Another internal heating agent now in use is a beam of exceedingly short wireless-waves, which has the same effect as diathermy. But these heating methods are applicable to very few diseases, for, on the whole, human tissues are more easily damaged by heat than are those of bacteria.

The other standard method of killing bacteria is to subject them to the action of chemicals. Almost as soon as bacteria were seriously studied it was found that hundreds of chemicals poisoned them with great ease. These disinfectants, as they were called, might be simple inorganic chemicals such as chloride of lime, iodine, mercuric chloride, or again organic derivatives such as formaldehyde, phenol (carbolic acid), cresol, etc. These were extremely useful in destroying bacteria, but all of them were general protoplasmic poisons — that is to say, substances which put a stop to the life-process, as soon as they came into contact with any sort of living matter. Naturally efforts were made to destroy bacteria in the body by injecting or administering disinfectants, but the result of all experiments was to show that there was no curative effect even when the dose was so great that the proportion of disinfectant in the tissues was large enough to have killed the bacteria had they been subjected to its action in the test-tube. Presumably these disinfectants either failed to enter the parts of the animal's tissues where the bacteria were ensconced, or, if they did so, they attached themselves to the tissues and not the bacteria. These results caused a certain discouragement among those who sought such remedies. Yet there were two facts which promised success, for there were two diseases, known to be parasitic, which could be cured by administering drugs. These were malaria, for which quinine was a specific, and syphilis, which was, apparently at least, cured by administering mercury compounds. As our knowledge of the nature of malaria became clearer it was proved that quinine, despite its harmlessness to human tissues, did in fact kill the malaria parasite at certain stages of its life-cycle. Yet it cured no other disease and it seemed as if there was some specific affinity between quinine and malaria-parasites. Thus it seemed reasonable to suppose that for other parasites there might be specific poisons, could we but find them. But how were we to look for them? There was not even the faintest hint of the mechanism by which quinine did its work — and at first there was nothing whatever to guide us in selecting chemicals to be tried out in experiments. And such, to-day, is the host of known chemicals, that if one hundred pathologists could each test one of them every week, they would not be finished in a century. Indeed, it is safe to say that since totally new organic chemicals are being produced at the rate of hundreds per month, it is quite unlikely that the therapeutic effects of all chemicals will ever be tried out.

Yet a great deal of progress has been made. For almost every protozoal disease (pp. 89-101) an efficient, if not perfect, curative drug has been found, and several of the worst bacterial diseases have been robbed of three-quarters of their terrors. The virus diseases, with one or two doubtful exceptions, still defy our efforts.

The problem may be stated thus: *'To find a drug which will reach the parasite in the tissues and will kill it with the minimum of danger and inconvenience to the patient.'*

The first condition rules out all the substances which combine with all kinds of protoplasm generally, and all highly reactive substances, such as chloride of lime, or permanganates. None of these can reach the parasite, for they combine with the proteins in the bloodserum, etc., long before they arrive at the scene of action. The next condition is that the drug should kill the parasite: to this end it must combine with some substance within it. It must not on the other hand kill the patient, so it must not combine with any essential substance in us. So really we need some not too reactive chemical which will combine with something in the parasite but not with anything in ourselves. We have, unfortunately, extremely little knowledge about the complex chemical substances in either parasite or man: so our search has to be largely irrational — guided, that is to say, by trial and error, based on previous experience.

We have, however, one guiding rule — the fact that substances which are chemically alike are usually therapeutically alike. So if we can find a chemical which incommodes the parasite to even a small extent, we can make a large number of its chemical relations in the lively hope that one of them may prove to be effective poison to the germ. The power to make entirely new chemical substances similar to, yet different from, a known substance, is the central feature of modern research on drugs. If we are to understand the story of the development of modern drugs we must see how this method came into being.

The arts and sciences of pharmacy and medicine probably sprang from the conscious recognition that poisonous plants, avoided even by animals, might be used as poisons or drugs. At or before the dawn of civilization medicines were prepared by pounding and boiling mixtures of herbs, and by the first century A. D. the chemist possessed most of the fundamental technique which sufficed to make the discoveries of the next seventeen hundred years. The idea of separating a crude drug into a small active part and a larger inert residue arose about the period of the Renaissance. In the seventeenth and eighteenth centuries the idea of a 'pure substance' came into being, and pure substances began to be extracted from familiar drugs. Thus from opium, the coagulated milky juice of certain types of poppy, there was extracted in 1807 a crystalline substance called morphine, which, unlike the original opium, could not be separated by physical processes such as recrystallization or distillation into any simpler substances, though chemical processes would, of course, break it down into other chemical substances. As time went on a number of pure substances were separated from plant drugs, e.g. strychnine from nux vomica, quinine from cinchona bark, etc.

On the other hand, chemists had for centuries recognized the possibility of making totally new drugs which had never existed until man began to take a hand in the work of creation. Calomel, Glauber salt,[1] tartar emetic, ether, chloroform, iodine, bismuth subnitrate, are examples of drugs which did not exist in any form, pure or impure, until the chemist, ancient or modern, found out how to make them. These substances are, however, of very simple chemical constitution, and had it not been for the rise of organic chemistry, the discovery of valuable drugs would very soon have ceased.

Organic chemistry is the chemistry of the compounds of the element carbon. Carbon differs from all the other chemical elements in that it forms a far greater number of compounds than any other element. All living things are largely composed of compounds of carbon—organic compounds, as we commonly call them. The behavior of these carbon compounds is so governed by laws which we have to some extent at least, been able to ascertain.

Systematic organic chemistry is entirely based on the idea of atoms and molecules. Everyone, to-day, is familiar with the idea of the atom, but some of us are not so sure about the molecule. If we consider a quantity of any pure substance —sugar, aspirin, epsom salts, chalk, choloroform, and so forth—we can obviously divide that quantity in half. But chemists and physicists believe, on very strong evidence, that these substances are not infinitely divisible, but that if it were possible to go on dividing time after time, a stage would

---

[1] This does exist in nature, but was first prepared artificially.

be reached when any further division would result in making a new substance. The smallest
particle of aspirin which could exist is called the
molecule of aspirin. If that molecule were split
into smaller parts the parts would not be aspirin,
but something else. Every pure substance, in
fact, is a mass of precisely similar molecules. So
if you ask: What is aspirin? the most precise answer is: It is the stuff which has molecules of the
pattern shown in Fig. 2. Molecules are made
up of atoms, which are the smallest particles of
chemical elements. Now, if we pick organic
compound to bits in the laboratory we find that
they are generally made up of carbon, hydrogen,
oxygen, very commonly nitrogen and sulphur,
and less commonly other elements. So the molecules of organic compounds must be built up of
atoms of carbon, hydrogen, oxygen, nitrogen, sulphur, etc., or some of these.

The organic chemists have spent a century on
finding out the patterns of atoms which make up
the molecules of various chemicals. They began
to clear up their ideas about these by the eighteen-
sixties, and to use them effectively from the
'seventies onward; to-day, when we know the
size and shape of atoms, they are able to map
out these patterns with the utmost accuracy and
clarity.

The atoms, which are the component parts of

the molecules, behave, for the chemist's purposes, as if they were tiny, hard spheres[1] from 1/750,-000,000 to about 1/50,000,000 of an inch in diameter. Each atom can link itself to a limited but well-defined number of other atoms and the points of linkage are at certain fixed angles to each other. We can, therefore, draw quite legitimate models of molecules and deduce from them a great deal about the manner in which substances having such molecules are likely to behave.

The process by which an organic chemist takes a natural substance — let us say nicotine —

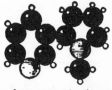

Black spheres represent carbon atoms.
Shaded spheres represent nitrogen atoms.
White spheres represent hydrogen atoms.

FIG. 1. Atom pattern of nicotine.

and deduces from the things he can do with it in the laboratory that its atom pattern must be that shown below, is impossible to explain without writing a textbook of organic chemistry; but, for the present, we may say that he can deduce the atom-patterns of the molecules of most substances which are not too complex. A few sub-

[1] The organic chemist's 'atom' is the territory around the physicist's atom which another atom cannot enter. Its internal arrangement of electron-shells, nucleus, etc., does not concern him: so although an atom is mostly empty space, he can treat it without error as a hard, solid sphere.

stances, notably the proteins, which are the stuff of living matter, still puzzle him. These, which have three thousand or more atoms in the molecule, might well baffle him, but even here he has some idea of the general plan on which such molecules are built up.

The atom pattern is not usually expressed by a model or a picture. For the convenience of printers and readers they are expressed as chemical formulæ. In these a capital letter (or pair of letters) is put in place of each atom and lines show which

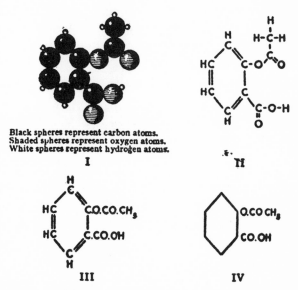

Black spheres represent carbon atoms.
Shaded spheres represent oxygen atoms.
White spheres represent hydrogen atoms.

I

II

III   IV

Fig. 2. Diagram of structure and chemical formulae of aspirin.

atoms are attached to which. Readers would not thank me for a complete exposition of chemical formulae—suffice it, then, to say that they are compact conventionalized ways of putting down atom-patterns on paper. Thus the atom pattern of aspirin is shown in Fig. 2, I. The chemical formula can be expressed as in II, or, more briefly, as III or IV. The systematic names of organic compounds are so designed to tell their formulæ to one who knows the key. Thus the drug sold under the original trade name of aspirin can be called by the organic chemist, acetylsalicyclic acid, or if we wish to be very concise, orthoacetoxyphenylcarboxylic acid — a name which tells the chemist the formula of the drug. The existence of several alternative nomenclatures does not generally confuse the organic chemist, but is troublesome to the doctor. The climax of absurdity is reached with the comparatively simple drug usually called sulphanilamide (p. 128). This has been given two or three reasonable ways of expressing its chemical title.

Atoms cannot be built up into molecules of any pattern we choose. There are certain well-defined groupings which persist through most of the chemical changes which a substance can undergo. The organic chemist has to-day a very fair idea of what is a possible atom-pattern and what is not, and he has collected and systematized an enormous number of tricks-of-the-trade, by which he can try to make a substance with molecules of any given reasonable specification. There is still plenty in the behavior of carbon compounds that is not understood, and, consequently, the building of a new substance to a specified formula is a matter for the exercise, not merely of the logical application of rules, but great ingenuity and technical skill. Some such problems prove highly resistant, thus no one has yet synthesized quinine, morphine, or (probably) cane-sugar, though the first of these problems has been worked on for eighty-four years at least. On the other hand, indigo, cocaine, glucose, were synthesized from simpler substances quite soon after their formulæ were known with certainty.

The art of synthesizing new compounds to order began to flourish exceedingly at just about the period when bacteria came into prominence. To a great extent money was at the bottom of it. In 1856 Perkin, in trying to make quinine, hit upon mauve, the first aniline dye. This discovery was a long way ahead of its time. In 1856 no one knew exactly what was the structure of the aniline molecule, far less that of the dye. But it was very soon evident that there was money in these dyes, and therefore in organic chemistry, theoretical and industrial. Perkin did not want to spend his life as a manufacturer, and in 1874 sold out his business and returned to research work in organic chemistry. The pursuit of synthetic dyes was soon taken up by the Germans and, although in the last two decades their supremacy has been assailed, they remain to this day the world's foremost organic chemists, in industry and research alike.

Dye-stuff materials—and most synthetic drugs —are more or less distantly derived from benzene. They contain one or more groups of six carbon atoms, arranged in a ring, which hangs together through the most elaborate chemical changes. The structure of this fundamental ring-group was worked out in 1865. This really started synthetic organic chemistry on its tremendous modern career. By 1875 most of its fundamental problems had been worked out, and an ever-increasing flood of new compounds was launched upon the world. Dyes, and of course the chemicals needed to make dyes, were the first of these products. The synthetic dye-industry went through a long stage, 1856-1874, when only a few products were made. But as organic chemistry developed, the power of research began to tell, and between 1874 and 1878 Germany gave the world a series of such coloring matters as it had never dreamed of — eosine, methylene blue, malachite green — which incidentally gave us valuable stains for the study of bacteria. In the 'eighties came artificial indigo and the azo-dyestuffs. This new type of manufacture could not be conducted without a large staff of trained chemists, not easy to find in the 'eighties. The Germans realized the need for expert personnel far more clearly than did the British, consequently the manufacture of dyes and fine chemicals drifted into their hands. The manufacture of drugs required the same type of men, materials, technique, and plant as the manufacture of dyes; so when the idea of synthetic drugs came to the fore it was in Germany that most of the work was done; and the manufacture of these drugs was, for a time, almost a

German monopoly.

The search for synthetic drugs seems at first to have centered on quinine. This drug is extracted from the bark of the cinchona three, a native of South America. The trees are now mostly grown in Java. The bark contains only 2 to 3 per cent of quinine and the preparation of the pure drug is fairly costly. Thus natural quinine can never be cheap, and even to-day in the largest wholesale transactions it costs about 70 cents an ounce. On the other hand, the demand for it is enormous, because a great part of the population of the tropics is infected with malarial fever. A synthetic quinine substitute which could be made cheaply would therefore be very valuable; to-day we can make at least two efficient synthetic substitutes (pp. 96, 97), but not, unfortunately, at a cost which would enable them to be supplied to the three hundred millions who need them. It was soon found that by breaking up quinine by various chemical means a liquid called quinoline was obtained. In 1879-1880 there was discovered a synthetic process by which this could be made cheaply and without using quinine. So naturally the chemists thought: 'Here is the root-substance of quinine: it may well be that some compound of it will prove to have the same effects as quinine itself.' In 1882 O. Fischer produced a simple quinoline compound, 'kairine,' which did, in fact, lower the temperature of a fevered person as quinine does. But it was not an antimalarial and, worst of all, it was decidedly poisonous. Then the

oddest thing happened. Knorr thought that he
could build up a drug with a molecule of the
quinoline atom-pattern from two other common
chemicals, acetoacetic ester and phenylhydrazine.
These, he found, duly reacted together and produced the new compound. This proved to be a
most useful drug: it decreased neuralgic pains,
much as aspirin does: it lowered the body temperature vigorously — but when its formula was
worked out it proved to have not the faintest re-
lationship to that of quinoline or quinine! The
discovery of this drug, which was called *antipyrine,* is a fine example of the way in which
scientific men work for one thing and find another.
The drug was of no use against malaria, but is
still in use in medicine as an antipyretic and anti-
neuralgic. Attempts were then made to find something better than antipyrine, and another drug
pyramidone, still more powerful, but also more
dangerous, was added to the doctor's armament.

In 1886 it was discovered that aniline itself
(which is highly poisonous) and a very simple
chemical acetanilide, had the same sort of effect
on the body as antipyrine. Acetanilide was a very
cheap substance, which antipyrine was not, so a
great deal of research was done in the hope of
finding something chemically like it, but free
from some of its defects, i.e. a tendency to damage
the blood-cells. So the chemists set to work to
prepare variants of it: that is to say, drugs with an
atom-pattern, in outline like that of acetanilide,
but differing in details. This idea of varying the

atom-pattern slightly in order to get a slightly different substance had become familiar in the dye industry, for it was well known that there were certain broad features of the general pattern of the molecules that gave the dyeing properties, while small alterations in the atom-pattern would alter the shade of the color. Accordingly the chemists altered the molecule of acetanilide and made a large number of similar substances having the same general effect on the body, but each having certain advantages or disadvantages. Only two survive in common use — acetanilide itself, used in headache powders, cold cures, etc., and phenacetin. The tow formulæ show the common feature of the pattern, the aniline group.

ANILINE

ACETANILIDE   PHENACETIN

It became apparent that there was generally a family resemblance between the molecules of drugs that affected the body in the same fashion, and in the years 1886-1889 this idea was worked out by Baumann and Kast for a very useful group of sleep-producing drugs, which still form a part of the physician's equipment. They found they could make a great many different drugs, all of which had molecules containing the group of atoms

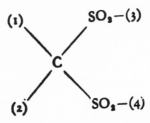

to which were attached various other groups of atoms at the points (1), (2), (3), (4). If one or more of these added groups was the 'ethyl' group, the drug was a hypnotic, and the more of these groups that were present the stronger was the effect. A good example is trional:

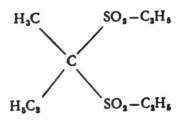

This research went far to fix the idea of finding an active substance and altering it to make it as effective as possible, but it did not give us any hint of how we were to look for new types of

active substances among the tens of thousands of
organic chemicals then known, and to this day we
are still almost as badly off in this respect. Between 1890 and 1910 an enormous number of
very useful drugs were made by the organic
chemist. Known to most people are acetanilide
(used in headache powders), aspirin, phenacetin,
sulphonal, veronal, luminal, heroin; actually sev-
eval hundred such drugs had been put on the
market, though comparatively few have survived
the test of time. None of these drugs were able
to *cure* any disease nor were they intended to do
so. Drugs, in fact, are generally not intended to
act on diseased tissues at all, but on healthy ones.
Codeine relieves a cough, but it does so, not by
restoring the inflamed membranes of the throat to
normality, but by deadening the sensitiveness of
the nerves which transmit its complaints. Digitalis
does not mend the damaged valves of the heart,
but it causes the still healthy heart muscle to act
in a more orderly fashion. The new synthetic
drugs which came into use between 1885 and
1910 were useful aids to the physician, for he
could use them to relieve symptoms of a disease,
and so diminish the strain on the body, thereby
increasing its resistance to the disease; but although the doctors did not advertise the fact to
their patients, they realized well enough that no
drugs went to the root of a germ-disease, the
progress of which could be arrested only by killing the germs — protozoa, bacteria, or virus —
or by destroying their toxins. In the discovery and

use of drugs which have this power resides the new science of Chemotherapy.

The enormous complication of our civilization is perhaps nowhere better shown than in the synthetic drug industry. Almost the simplest of these drugs is aspirin, brought into use about 1900, and now to be found in every medicine chest, affording as it does a means of alleviating the two commonest kinds of pain, headache and toothache. A century ago we took laudanum — a solution of opium in alcohol — as a remedy for toothache. It was pretty effective, but, of course, was a powerful poison and a serious habit-former. It was made by incising the heads of opium-poppies, scraping off the half-solidified juices, drying these, and moulding the product into lumps. This gave opium: by extracting the active portion with alcohol one obtained laudanum. Quite a domestic affair. Some natives of Asia made the opium by hand. Somebody shipped it to England, and the druggist made it into landanum at the back of his shop.

Now compare the processes needed to make a tablet of aspirin. Its raw materials are coal and air and water, but if we include materials used in the manufacture but not appearing in the final product we may add limestone, salt, and sulphur. None of these is very recondite: but it is the habit of our civilization to build a few simple materials into a myriad complex and diverse products. Our tablet of aspirin involves the labor of thousands of men. The miner hews coal, the railways carry it, the gas-works distill it and obtain tar. Refineries distill crude benzol from this. The chemical works extract pure benzene from this and perform seven separate chemical operations on it to make it into salicylic acid. These operations need pure sulphuric acid, whose manufacture from American sulphur is a vast industry in itself; lime, involving the quarrymen and the modern large-scale lime-kilns, which we see in the Midlands; soda, the making of which is another great industry.

The salicylic acid has to be combined with acetyl chloride to make aspirin. To make this we start with coke and lime and electrical power and make calcium carbide; from this we obtain acetylene which with steam and air can be persuaded to form acetic acid and ultimately acetyl chloride. This, combined with the salicylic acid, gives aspirin. The aspirin once made is elaborately crystallized to purify it, and then made into tablets. Roughly speaking, *nineteen* chemical processes are needed, not counting those required to manufacture the chemicals involved in the making of the aspirin but not entering into the final product — and aspirin is perhaps the simplest of synthetic drugs. We may well realize that it is not the research chemist alone who has given us these drugs, but that their availability depends on a gigantic industrial system extending over the whole world. Such a breakdown of our modern civilization as might be caused by a long series of devastating wars would not, in all probability, involve a necessary disappearance of science, for there would be books and men to read them. But it would mean the loss of nearly all the benefits of science for most of its achievements can be fulfilled only through the co-operation, conscious or otherwise, of the greater part of the world's industries.

CHAPTER IV

THE RISE OF CHEMOTHERAPY

*Work of Ehrlich on trypanosomiasis — Atoxyl —
Salvarsan (606) — Tropical disease —
Hook-worm — Bilharziasis — Malaria —
Kala-azar — Amœbic dystentery — Sleep-
ing sickness — Yaws — Leprosy.*

CHEMOTHERAPY, the radical cure of parasitic diseases by drugs, owes its origin mainly
to Paul Ehrlich, a Jew born in Silesia. He was
at once bacteriologist, organic chemist, and medical man. He had long been interested in aniline
dyes, as was natural, since he grew up in the
period when the dye-industry was new. He had
observed the staining of bacteria by dyes and
reflected on it; and he came to think of a poison as
something analogous to a dye. A dye may attach
itself to some particular textile fibre such as the
wool-fibre and cannot thereafter be washed out
of it, although the same dye may be readily
washed away from cotton or linen or any other
material. So Ehrlich thought that a poison was
something that attached itself, indelibly, so to
speak, to the living cell. He visualized the possibility of finding poisons which would attach
themselves to the parasite's cell, but not to the
cells of the tissue of its host; and, naturally
enough, he sought for such poisons in the class
of dyes.

89

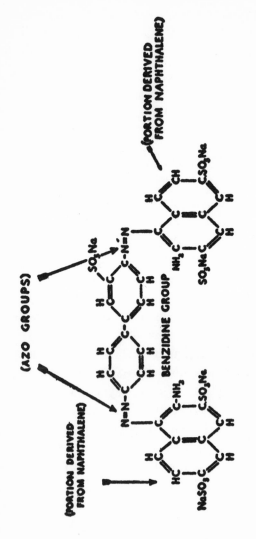

FORMULA OF TRYPAN RED

A number of tropical diseases are caused by protozoa called *trypanosomes* which are conveyed to men and animals by the agency of biting flies, in particular the notorious tsetse. In men they cause sleeping-sickness, the scourge of much of tropical Africa. In cattle they cause Nagana cattle plague, which makes it impossible to keep many types of hoofed animals throughout a great part of Africa. Ehrlich studied the effect of dyes on those parasites. In 1906 he discovered trypan violet, followed in 1907 by trypan red, and later trypan blue and naga red. These were very complex dyes derived from naphthalene. They were, on the whole, pretty effective, and a series of injections would apparently kill all the trypanosomes in an affected animal. These dyes were too poisonous to retain their popularity and they have now dropped out of use. But they definitely proved that chemotherapy was a reasonable possibility. Ehrlich continued his work and tried a new line of research. Arsenic is a very general poison. Could it, he wondered, be so bound up in an organic compound that it would stick to the tissues of the parasite and not the host Ehrlich and his co-workers synthesized a great number of arsenical organic compounds. In 1907 they produced atoxyl, which promised remarkable results and did cure many thousands of cases of sleeping-sickness. But it had the very serious effect of sometimes attacking the optic nerve and causing blindness: several variations on atoxyl were tried, but none were entirely satisfactory.

The first real triumph of chemotherapy was Ehrlich and Hata's discovery in the year 1910 of the famous arsenical drug '606'.

Its full chemical title is 3:3'—diamino—4:4'—dyhydroxy-arseno-benzene, and its formula is shown below:

FORMULA OF SALVARSAN (ARSPHENAMINE)
"As"DENOTES AN ATOM OF ARSENIC

The drug has borne many different names. Salvarsan was its first title; it is sold by many firms under different denominations, but its official B.P. denomination is now arsphenamine. This drug had the most astonishing effect on the common and extremely serious disease of syphilis. In favorable cases the injection of the drug might cause all visible sign of the disease to vanish in a fortnight, and it seemed at first as if Ehrlich's ideal of a drug which would destroy the whole host of parasites by a single or a few doses had been realized. This proved to be too hopeful, for a small proportion of parasites always remained unscathed, and we now know that it is necessary to give a course of injections of an arsenical drug and of a preparation of heavy metal, formerly mercury, but now usually bismuth, for a period of 1½-2 years. Arsphenamine has been superseded by neo-arsphenamine, introduced by Ehrlich two years later, and by sulpharsphenamine. The injection of one of these drugs is still the standard treatment for syphilis, and there is no question but that they have enormously increased the probability of cure and have greatly decreased the number of infectious syphilitics capable of spreading the disease. The best proof of the efficacy of the treatment is given by the number of babies dying each year from hereditary syphilis. Before 1920 this ranged around 100-1500, now it is about 120. Salvarsan created enormous interest and its high success had the result of concentrating much more research on the finding of new chemotherapeutic remedies. The progress of the work falls into two main periods; the years 1910-1935, during which remedies were found for most of the tropical diseases, and the period since 1935 in which drugs active against bacteria have been studied.

It is not easy for the stay-at-home American to realize the tragedy of tropical disease, and its paralyzing effect upon the human race. Vast populations numbered in hundreds of millions are riddled with disease. In most tropical regions of the world every person has suffered to a greater or less extent from malaria, and in damp, tropical regions 80 per cent of these suffer also from hook-worm. The death-rate from these diseases, from kala-azar, sleeping-sickness, dysentery, make our European mortalities look puny; worse still, most of these give rise to chronic infections and so cause whole populations to suffer from permanent ill-health. It is interesting to conjecture whether the tropical races might have had the energy and driving force of the temperate, if they had not suffered from the permanent debility induced by chronic diseases.

These tropical diseases are mostly caused either by comparatively large parasites such as flatworms, or by protozoa (pp. 27-28), and there are not many exclusively tropical bacterial diseases. Most of these diseases were in the past practically incurable; they did not, of course, necessarily cause death, but if they did not, the patient usually remained to some extent infected and more or less ill throughout his life. Against nearly all of these diseases there are now effective chemotherapeutic remedies; the difficulty is to provide them in adequate quantity and to assure their use. At present there are perhaps 300,000,000 people actively suffering from malaria. Most of these people are at a very low level of subsistence, and cannot pay for medical treatment. To give them even five grains of quinine a day would cost more than $750,000,000 a year — nor indeed are there cinchona trees enough in the world to provide a fraction of this quinine; so, for the most part, they go untreated. Even when free treatment for a disease is available it is not easy to persuade simple people that they need it before they are *in extremis*. It is not enough to discover and pay for an effective drug: an elaborate health service must be provided, and, unless it can compel patients to be treated, it will not very greatly reduce the mass of ill-health.

We may start by devoting a word or two to hook-worm disease, which affects perhaps 80 to 90 per cent of the native populations in moist, tropical countries and induces a chronic state of weakness and ill-health. This disease can be cured by poisoning the 'worms' inside the intestine by carbon tetrachloride or hexyl-resorcinol. This is a sort of chemtherapy, but it differs from the other cases we shall consider in that the worms reside in the intestines and are therefore, strictly speaking, outside the body. Another disease caused by larger parasites is bilharziasis—known affectionately in Egypt as Bill Harris. This affects some ten million people in Egypt alone, and probably many times more in other hot climates. It is a serious illness having an appreciable mortality. Its cause is infestation by flat-worms which inhabit the bladder, liver, and spleen. These creatures have the curious life-history which characterizes most flat-worms. One stage of their life-history is carried out in a human being, the other in a water-snail. Eggs are laid by the adult worms in the human body and pass out with the urine or fæces. They hatch to a larva which enters the body of a water-snail, develops in it to a second type of larva which escapes into the water and bores through the skin of any person with whom it may come in contact, and in his tissues it develops once more into a adult flat-worm. The conditions for the spread of the disease are (1) a warm climate, (2) contamination of water with urine and fæces, (3) a human population which commonly enters the water. It is at present impossible to teach hygiene to primitive populations; so the disease continues.

In 1917 Christopherson discovered that tartar emetic (a compound of antimony) when injected into the blood cures the disease, and since then millions of people have been treated. Tartar emetic, however, has the objection that a long course of treatment is required and a great many patients give up before they are cured; moreover, it can be rather painful. Since that time several other drugs have been introduced, one of the best being fouadin, a complex organic compound of antimony. This may cure some 60 to 80 per cent of patients. The improvement over the conditions which prevailed before 1917 is tremendous, but none of the compounds as yet available are effective enough to stamp out the disease from a whole population.

The problem of malaria is a tremendous one. The disease affects some three hundred million people, and certainly causes several million deaths every year. We have already discussed the ways in which it is transmitted and have seen that it is not always possible to stamp out the transmitting agent — the mosquito. Malaria may have been treated by chemotherapy from time immemorial in Peru, where cinchona bark was a native remedy, but the first recorded case of its successful use is supposed to have been the curing of a Spanish corregidor by cinchona bark in 1630. Two years later it was introduced into Europe. Cinchona bark remained the standard remedy for malaria for some two hundred years. In 1820 its active principal, quinine, was extracted, and this has remained our standby in malarial cases. Most white people in the malarial regions of the tropics take five grains of quinine every day: this does not seem to prevent malaria altogether, but it keeps it within reasonable proportions. Quinine is a true chemotherapeutic remedy. It kills the malaria parasite in the asexual stages of its life-history, and it will usually cure malaria if it is persevered with.

It has the rare advantage of being almost without poisonous properties: in fact, it is thought that no one has ever been killed by a single dose of quinine, however enormous, which is decidedly more than can be said for its synthetic rivals. Two such drugs, both very active, have been brought into use in curing malaria. They are *plasmoquine* and *atebrin*. These drugs kill the malaria parasite quite successfully, and plasmoquine has the advantage of killing the sexual forms of the parasite, which quinine itself does not affect. But both drugs are very expensive and both are rather poisonous, that is to say, the dose needed to kill the parasites is undesirably near that needed to kill the patient. Quinine still remains the standard antimalarial; if some organic chemist could find a way to synthesize it really cheaply he would confer a gigantic benefit on humanity. But I do not anticipate an immediate success. The atom-pattern of quinine is a very peculiar one and does not look at all promising for the chemist.

Hook-worm, bilharziasis, and malaria, are tolerated the more easily by the human race because a great many of those who suffer from them are, for most of the time, well enough to go about their business; but this is not the case with all tropical diseases, for among them are some of the most disabling and fatal of human ills.

Perhaps the most striking success of chemo-therapy has been the treatment of kala-azar, a protozoal disease transmitted, we know to-day, by the bites of a minute sand-fly. This fever devastated Assam and Bengal at the beginning of this century, and reduced the population of the affected areas by some 30 per cent. About 90 per cent of the patients died after a long-drawn-out illness. In 1915 it was found that antimony compounds were an effective cure. Tartar emetic was injected into the veins of the patients, and instead of 90 per cent dying, over 90 per cent recovered. Other synthetic antimonial drugs, notably neostibosan, are probably better and less unpleasant than tartar emetic, but the latter is effective and not expensive, so it is still much in use. It is difficult to estimate the number of lives this treatment has saved. Several thousands of cases are treated yearly, and three hundred thousand lives would be a low estimate of the total rescued from a slow death. It is interesting to reflect on the fact that the average American has not even heard of this gigantic triumph of science over death.

Amœbic dysentery is a tropical disease in which the wall of the intestines is attacked and damaged by an amœba — a simple form of protozoon. A remarkable cure for this intractable disease was found in the active principle of ipecacuanha root, known as emetine. The drug is, however, decidedly poisonous, and efforts have been made to find something which will kill the amœba more safely. A synthetic drug iodohydroxyquinolinesulphonic acid (known as chiniofon, yatren, etc.), has proved very successful in the less advanced cases, as also have some of the arsenical drugs — but the synthetic drugs are expensive and not over-reliable, and emetine remains the mainstay of treatment.

The disease of trypanosomiasis, or sleeping-sickness[1] has already been mentioned. It is caused by two protozoa, *Trypanosoma gambiense* and *rhodesiense*. It is a slow but very fatal disease leading finally to a state of bodily and mental breakdown, stupor and death. It has, as far as we know, always been prevalent in West Africa, but serious attention was drawn to it, when as a result of the opening of trade-routes from West Africa to Uganda it was introduced into the area around Lake Victoria Nyanza, an area inhabited by a population without natural immunity to its attack, and swarming with tsetse flies, which

[1] Not to be confused with the so-called 'sleepy sickness' or encephalitis lethargica.

transmit the disease by their bite. Some districts were almost depopulated. In one area the population fell from 56,000 to 13,000, and it is estimated that in all 200,000 East African natives died. The efforts of Ehrlich produced *atoxyl* (p. 91) in 1907. This cured a great number of cases but it was not altogether satisfactory, for while it killed the trypanosome, it sometimes attacked the patient's optic nerve and caused blindness. At present the drug chiefly relied on is an arsenical compound *tryparsamide* (p. 102). This accomplishes 75 to 80 per cent of cures. Another and very remarkable drug is Bayer 205 or Germanin, an exceedingly complicated chemical with the formula shown on p. 102. It was introduced in 1923. Its formula was not disclosed and the patents covering it were so vague and comprehensive that no one could deduce what it was. However, Fourneau arrived at the same drug and published the formula. The commercial system which allows such things to be kept secret criticizes itself. The drug is extraordinarily specific. If the portentous atom pattern shown on p. 102 is altered by merely removing the two CH_3 groups shown in darker type, the whole of its activity is lost! The —CH_3 group in general has no special active properties and the reason why this particular pattern of atoms is able to link up to something in the trypanosome is wholly obscure. Germanin is very successful in early cases, but once the nervous system is affected it seems to do little good.

Recently another interesting line of research

has come into prominence. When trypanosomes were grown in artificial culture, they were found to use up relatively enormous quantities of glucose — a sugar always and necessarily present in the blood. So it seemed possible that the administration of a drug which would lower the proportion of sugar in the blood might prevent their development. One such drug, *synthalin,* proved to have the effect desired. This preliminary success led to the investigation of similar drugs and some extremely promising ones have been discovered. But, oddly enough, their effect appears to have nothing to do with the lowering of the blood-sugar, but to be an entirely specific effect! Great hopes are entertained that some of these, such as diamidinostilbene, will solve the problem of human trypanosome diseases. Preliminary experiments show great promise, but the drugs have not yet (1940) been tried out on the large scale.

Every effort has been made to stamp out the disease. So far no very satisfactory way of attempting this has been found. Tsetse flies are very hard to eliminate, for though they are slow breeders, they inhabit an enormous area of country and have no habits which might make them specially vulnerable. There has been a belief that the trypanosomes harbored by big game, e.g. antelopes, are carried by tsetse flies to man, but it seems unlikely that these species of trypanosome cause sleeping-sickness in man. If so, we cannot stamp out sleeping-sickness by killing off game.

MOLECULE OF TRYPARSAMIDE

FORMULA OF ATEBRIN

THE FORMULA OF GERMANIN (BAYER 205)

The most hopeful course is to stamp out the disease in men. In Bahr-El-Ghazal, a large province in the Southern Sudan, the whole population was examined and all sleeping-sickness cases collected into separate communities and treated. In this way the disease was almost entirely stamped out, for no patients were left to infect the tsetse flies. How far such a course is possible in other parts of Africa time will doubtless show.

Spectacular successes have been scored with two diseases — yaws and relapsing fever — which are caused by parasites somewhat resembling those which cause syphilis. Both these diseases are very quickly cured by the same agents as cure syphilis, e.g. neo-arsphenamine.

Yaws is a disease which, even untreated, has but a small death-rate — about $2\frac{1}{2}$ per cent. It is characterized by the formation of large, disfiguring sores, often on the face, which in the course of years may give place to deep corroding ulcers. The drug acts in a most dramatic fashion and the cures it produces has converted some native populations to a tardy belief in European medicine.

Finally, the dread and ancient disease of leprosy has been assailed, not by a wholly new synthetic drug, but by a purified and modified form of chaulmoogra oil, a plant product which has been known in India for centuries as a remedy. This oil was not, however, of much value until the plan of injecting it into the muscles was evolved. The injection of the crude oil was so painful that patients would not accept the treatment; but of recent years a pure chemical compound, ethyl chaulmoograte, has been made from the oil, and can be safely injected. This cures 40 to 50 per cent of the victims of this hitherto hopeless disease. But here again the difficulty is to find lepers, for until native patients begin to suffer seriously they do not realize they are lepers, or if they do so, they are not unduly worried. There are still some two hundred thousand lepers in Nigeria alone. The figure for the whole world must be well above the million mark.

It appears then that we possess the scientific means of curing most tropical diseases. If England were miraculously transported to the Congo there is no doubt that we should wipe out almost all tropical disease from it in ten years, even if we wiped out the jungle and the fauna in doing it. But as things stand, we are sorry to see millions of natives perishing, but we are not sorry enough to put ourselves about it. And until the rich nations who draw wealth from the tropics put more of it back into health services, tropical disease must continue. It is, in a way, a thankless task, for in most instances, the native does not want to be treated, if it is to be any inconvenience to him. Are we justified in forcing health upon him by compelling him to be medically examined, to receive injections, and so forth? It is very hard to decide, especially in the case of races which are too advanced to be treated paternally, yet not advanced enough to have acquired a civilized attitude to hygiene.

CHAPTER V

PRONTOSIL

*Gerard Domagk—Discovery of a chemotherapeutic
dye—Prontosil—Testing of drugs on animals and human beings—Activity of drug
against streptococci — Diseases caused by
streptococci—Sulphanilamide—The conquest
of puerperal fever.*

WHILE the remarkable successes we have re-
counted were being obtained in the treatment of protozoal diseases, no appreciable results
were obtained in the chemotherapy of diseases
caused by bacteria. Work was done on the subject, but since negative results are commonly
left unpublished there is little record remaining.
The great successes in the drug treatment of bacterial disease that have been attained since 1935
are due primarily to the perseverance and genius
of Gerard Domagk.

Domagk is now only forty-six years of age. He
is a German—a Brandenburger; he fought against
the Allies and was wounded in the war of 1914-
1918. After the war he took up the question of
the means by which the reticuloendothelial system
of the body kills the bacteria it takes from the
blood-stream (p. 52). He thought it must contain

some chemical substance which acted on the bacteria and, accordingly, he tried to extract this from the tissues in question, but without result. He then devoted himself to finding some synthetic drug which should have this destructive power. In 1927 he was appointed Director of Experimental Pathology and Bacteriology at the Elberfeld laboratories of the great firm of I. G. Farbenindustrie, of which Messrs. Bayer are a subsidiary.

What was there to guide him in his search for such a substance among the half-million known, and the perhaps infinite number of unknown, chemicals? Some types of chemical were obviously unsuitable as being physiologically inert, or, on the other hand, as being destructive to tissues in general. The most likely hint was given by Ehrlich's notion that dyes might be selective poisons. Certainly the latter's trypan red and blue had had some success, and other workers had found that certain azo-dyes (those containing a group of two linked nitrogen atoms —N=N—) had some power of killing bacteria.

Domagk was primarily a pathologist and bacteriologist and not a chemist. So he collaborated with two organic chemists, Mietzsch and Klarer, who at his instance prepared a large number of these azo-dyes. Some of these proved to be disinfectants, that is to say, substances capable of killing bacteria outside the body, but this was not what he was seeking. In 1932, however, Domagk found that one of Mietzsch and Klarer's new dyes, when injected into mice which had been infected with streptococci, had a definite curative effect. This was a most significant discovery, for the streptococci were, of all bacteria, perhaps the most difficult to influence. No drugs affected them and serum treatment was of little use, probably because there are, in fact, some thirty strains of *streptococcus pyogenes* which are not rapidly distinguishable from each other and which all require different sera; and these, even when correctly selected and applied, are not usually of much avail. Consequently, the diseases caused by the more virulent strains of streptococci, which the body does not easily combat, had a high mortality. Especially was this the case with blood-poisoning, puerperal fever, and erysipelas in young children. A remedy for streptococcal infections was, therefore, a discovery of which the world stood in urgent need.

The molecule of the dye which first showed promise contained a grouping of atoms which the chemists call the *sulphonamide* group. It has the formula $SO_2 . NH_2$. Dye with this grouping in their molecules had been made as long ago as 1910 by Hoerlein, Dressel, and Kothe; at which period they were investigated, not because they might have medicinal properties, but because they adhered extremely firm to wool-fibre and were very fast to washing. This seemed at the time of Domagk's discovery a possible reason why they should adhere to the proteins of bacteria and so poison them: but in fact their effect on bacteria had nothing at all to do with their dyeing properties.   Perkin, in 1856, looked for the drug quinine, and found the first synthetic dye, mauve.

This discovery was only the first step in a gigantic research.   The new dye might be effective against streptococci: but was it the most effective of all such possible dyes?

The only way to find out was to make a great number of such dyes and try them out.   The synthesis of a new drug may be a very laborious task or fairly simple.   Most of the azo-dyes are not difficult to make, but they have to be very scrupulously purified before they can be tested, and moreover, the chemical formulæ of the products have to be established without doubt.   The workers of the Elberfeld laboratories set to work to synthesize as many dyes as possible, having in their structure a 'sulphonamide' or some similar group of atoms.   It soon became apparent that this power of causing the death of bacteria while in the tissues of an animal belonged to a large class of such dyes and not to one or two alone. More than 1,000 such compounds were made, many of which were highly active against streptococci in the bodies of test-animals — though, strange to relate, outside the body they were but feeble disinfectants.   In 1932 Mietzsch and Klarer prepared a new dye-stuff which proved to be the most effective of this multitude and which has since made a great noise in the medical world.   It was the hydro-chloride of a base whose chemical name is 4-sulphonamido-2', 4',-diaminoazobenzene, which formidable mouthful is an expression of the chemical formula:

When its usefulness was discovered it was given the more convenient trade-name of *prontosil*.

The medical world in general knew nothing about all this until 1935, though one or two Germanic clinicians were allowed to test the drug on human patients. It is said that Domagk felt the results to be too good to be true, and required to give the drug the most rigid tests before he published anything. The ordinary scientific worker cannot but feel, however, that these three years of secrecy were not in the best interests either of science or humanity: and he cannot but wonder whether they were not dictated by the commercial necessity of gaining a knowledge of the new group before commercial rivals could do so — a perfectly legitimate and almost necessary practice as long as such research is carried out almost exclusively by profit-earning corporations. Be that as it may, the year 1935 saw the launching of the new drug and the announcement from a dozen or more sources that it had an effect on streptococcal diseases which seemed at that time little less than miraculous.

At this point crops up a question which we should have asked before, namely: How do we assess the effectiveness of drugs? The testing of the curative powers of such drug requires perhaps even more skill than their synthesis. There are two chief stages in the trial, the test upon animals and those upon human patients. Anyone with normal views about the relative sanctity of human and animal life will see the need that the first test should be on animals. Almost all drugs are poisonous if taken in large enough doses and it is clear that the fatal dose cannot be ascertained by experiment on human beings.

But the testing of the effect of drugs on animals is beset with difficulties. The tests are carried out by bacteriologists or pathologists, usually in the laboratories of the chemical manufacturers, but sometimes at specialized institutions, such as the Lister Institute. It is necessary to use small and reasonably inexpensive animals which can be handled under laboratory conditions. Mice, rats, guinea-pigs, rabbits, etc., fulfil these conditions, but they differ quite considerably from human beings in their sensitiveness to attack by bacteria. Some bacteria will not infect mice at all, despite the fact that they may cause rapid and dangerous infections in man: such, for example, is the gonococcus. Fortunately, however, mice are rapidly killed by the β-hæmolytic streptococcus. It was found that mice injected with a suitable dose of these bacteria invariably died, while if they were given a certain

measured dose of prontosil they usually recovered.

The minimum quantity of the drug needed
to poison an average mouse of standard weight
was also determined, and it was then possible to
discover the 'therapeutic ratio' of the drug. If
the average weight of the drug required to kill
the mouse is fifty times greater than the average
weight needed to cure the mouse of the infection,
we say that the therapeutic ratio of the drug is
50. It is obviously desirable that this figure should
be as large as possible, the more so since a small
proportion of patients are likely to be exceptionally sensitive to the drug in question. From these
experiments a rough idea of the suitable dose
could also be obtained, for, roughly speaking,
if a man weighs three thousand times as much
as a mouse, he may expect to require a dose
about three thousand times as large.

The next stage was the testing of the drugs on
human patients. The ordinary practitioner cannot do this, for two things are desirable—a long
run of cases and the use of controls. The effectiveness of a treatment cannot be assessed by the
opinions of general practitioners who see its effect on their daily work. Statistics are required,
and these should be based on some numerically
measurable data. The best indicator of the value
of the treatment of a serious disease is the mortality — the percentage of the patients who die,
for there can be no two opinions as to whether
a patient is alive or dead. A better criterion in

diseases which have little or no mortality is the duration of the disease, the number of days the patient remains in hospital, or in bed, or with a high temperature, etc.

Let us suppose, then, that our test of a new drug shall be a comparison of the percentage of patients treated with it who recover, with the percentage of patients who recover when treated without it. This seems sound enough; yet two very important conditions must be fulfilled. Firstly a large number of patients must be studied: secondly, it must be certain that the treated patients and the untreated are similar people suffering from precisely the same type of disease.

First as to the number of patients. We want to find, by observation, the proportion of them which gets well. The difficulty of this can be illustrated by a simple experiment. Suppose you want to find the percentage of 'heads' that come down when a penny is tossed. You have no doubt, I am sure, that 'in the long run' the answer is 50 per cent. But if you try the experiment you will find that your result is not exactly 50 per cent, but that, generally speaking, the more times the penny is tossed the nearer to 50 per cent the proportion comes. The table on the following page shows the result of such an experiment.

Now suppose that we were dealing not with coins but with patients suffering from a disease which on a very long run would have 50 per cent mortality. The 'throws' now represent cases; the 'heads,' deaths, the 'tails,' recoveries; and the percentage of heads the mortality rate. If the doctor had been able to study only the first three cases, the mortality would have seemed to him to be 66.7 per cent; if the first ten cases, 30 per cent; if twenty cases, 45 per cent. By the time he had tested fifty cases he would have a pretty clear idea of the real mortality, though he would probably conclude that the mortality was

RESULT OF TOSSING A PENNY FIFTY TIMES

Number of throw	Result	Total Heads	% Heads	Number of throw	Result	Total Heads	% Heads
1	Head	1	100	26	Head	13	50
2	Head	2	100	27	Head	14	51.8
3	Tail	2	66.7	28	Head	15	53.6
4	Tail	2	50	29	Head	16	55.2
5	Tail	2	40	30	Tail	16	53.3
6	Tail	2	33.3	31	Tail	16	51.6
7	Head	3	42.9	32	Tail	16	50
8	Tail	3	37.5	33	Tail	16	48.5
9	Tail	3	33.3	34	Tail	16	47.0
10	Tail	3	30.0	35	Tail	16	45.7
11	Tail	3	27.3	36	Tail	16	44.4
12	Head	4	33.3	37	Head	17	46.0
13	Tail	4	30.8	38	Tail	17	44.8
14	Head	5	35.7	39	Head	18	46.1
15	Tail	5	33.3	40	Tail	18	45.0
16	Head	6	37.5	41	Head	19	46.4
17	Head	7	41.2	42	Tail	19	45.3
18	Head	8	44.4	43	Tail	19	44.2
19	Head	9	47.4	44	Head	20	45.4
20	Tail	9	45.0	45	Tail	20	44.4
21	Tail	9	42.9	46	Head	21	45.7
22	Tail	9	40.9	47	Head	22	46.8
23	Head	10	43.5	48	Head	23	47.9
24	Head	11	45.9	49	Tail	23	46.9
25	Head	12	48.0	50	Head	24	48.0

about 46 to 47 per cent. This departure from the true 50 per cent would be unimportant because mortality rates vary considerably from time to time and from place to place.

It is clear then that only in hospital practice can a sufficiently long series of cases be obtained. But even here there are difficulties. A penny remains the same, however long you go on tossing it, but a disease does not. Thus an epidemic usually begins with a high mortality-rate which slackens off as it dies out. Even diseases which do not run in very notable epidemics, e.g. pneumonia, vary greatly in their virulence; thus the mortality of pneumonia in the same month of two successive years might differ by 3 or 4 per cent. The virulence of bacteria varies, and so does the resistance of patients. So it is not always safe to compare the mortality of patients treated in one way at one time with that of those treated in anoher way at another time, for the illness may not be identical. The ideal method of testing is to treat with the drug every other patient entering a hospital until a hundred or more have received the drug and a hundred or more 'controls' have been treated without it. The use of controls is the only scientific method of testing, and although it may be very hard to withhold an apparently effective remedy from the untreated hundred, they will be no worse off than the thousands who went before them, and humanity as a whole will benefit from the certain knowledge gained. The results should then, apart from the unavoidable operations of chance, be strictly comparable. Even the operation of chance can be minimized, for a mathematical treatment will show whether the difference between the two series is significant, that is to say, too large to be expected from the operation of chance. Thus if 20 out of 100 treated patients and 45 out of 100 untreated patients died, this difference would be significant; but if 20 of 100 treated patients and 22 of 100 untreated patients died the figures would not be significant; for the next hundred tested might by mere chance show these figures reversed.

Medical men are not always too judicious about their reports, and so many remedies have been cried up on the strength of half a dozen cases that the profession has become skeptical about new ways of treatment. In the words of a famous physician, "Make haste to use a new remedy before it is too late."

Most of the reports on the new sulphonamide drugs are, however, beyond reproach. The series of cases are long and often controlled. For some of the rarer diseases a long series cannot be obtained. Reports concerning these must be treated with caution unless the mortality-rate with the drug is very different from that without. If, however, a disease is of such virulence that 95 per cent of its victims die, then a much shorter series of cases—say four recoveries and one death—will amount to good evidence of the effectiveness of the treatment. Thus even three or four successive recoveries in streptococcal meningitis would be impressive, for from this disease almost no one recovers.

It is easily seen then that the making and experimental testing of a new group of drugs can hardly be looked on as an isolated discovery of a single man, for it involves an enormous volume of work by dozens of research workers skilled in different aspects of the subject. The organic chemist, the analyst, the bacteriologist and pathologist, and the physician, all have to co-operate under the leadership of the director of research of the institution. It is clear, too, that this work is quite unsuitable for the single worker in his private laboratory or even for a small college or institute, for it is extremely difficult to arrange for the collaboration of all the experts whose servives are needed unless all are members of the same institution.

The study of the thousand or so drugs synthesized at Elberfeld seemed to show that all the effective ones contained in their molecules the groupings of atoms:

$$(1)\text{-}N\text{=}N\text{-}C \underset{\underset{(4)}{C}=\underset{(5)}{C}}{\overset{\overset{(2)\quad(3)}{C-C}}{\bigodot}} C\text{-}SO_2\text{-}N \overset{(6)}{\underset{(7)}{\diagup}}$$

To this skeleton other groupings were attached in the positions 1 to 7. Most of the resulting drugs were to some extent effective, but they varied in therapeutic power and in toxicity. On the

whole they proved to be remarkably inert in their
behavior to the human body and doses of several
grammes could be safely taken.   By 1935 it was
quite clear that prontosil was the best of these
drugs.   In that year Domagk published his results and for the first time the world had a remedy against *streptococcus pyogenes,* the β-hæmolytic streptococcus.   Actually this bacterium exists
in more than thirty strains, some of which are
more readily affected by the drug than others.
This bacterium has three chief effects on the human body: first, it produces a poison which destroys the red blood-cells and thus puts the blood
out of action: secondly, it has a great power of
invading the tissues, leading to rapid spread and
in some instances to infection of the whole blood-
stream; thirdly, it may cause red rashes on the
skin, as in erysipelas and scarlet fever.

Streptococci are almost ubiquitous, but the
type which causes our troubles is chiefly to be
found in the human throat and on the human
hand.   One person in fourteen or fifteen carries it
in the nose or throat and about one person in
twenty-seven carries it on the hands.   It is also
found in the dust of wards where cases of infection by it are being nursed, but not as a rule
in ordinary dust and dirt.   The prevalence of this
bacterium in the nose and throat is the chief reason
why those who are present at surgical operations
wear masks of gauze designed to arrest droplets
of saliva (p. 38).

The bacterium causes symptoms which depend

both on the virulence of the strain concerned and on the part of the body affected. So streptococcal invasion is classified into some fifteen diseases — nearly all serious.

The simplest case to consider is when the bacterium gains access to the body by way of a wound, as is likely to happen when a doctor cuts himself during a post-mortem, or may, though less probably, occur when any of us cuts himself with a dirty instrument, or infects a cut with bacteria from our own or someone else's throat.

If the bacterium multiplies in and about the wound and invades the surrounding tissues great swelling and redness and pain are produced together with grave illness. This condition is known as *cellulitis*. If the bacterium invades the bloodstream and multiplies therein it is know as *streptococcal septicæmia*. Both of these conditions are very serious and, indeed, streptococcal septicæmia — in lay terms blood-poisoning — has a mortality of round about 75 per cent — only one recovery in every four cases.

When a baby is born there is very commonly some degree of inner damage to the mother. This usually repairs itself without incident, but in about one case in six hundred the injury becomes infected with streptococci. This condition is called *puerperal fever*. It is very serious and about one in four of its victims die, which meant that every year, in England and Wales, for instance, before the introduction of these drugs, about one thousand of our most valuable assets —

healthy mothers — were lost from this cause, and
this in spite of the most rigid precautions aimed
at excluding the bacterium.

Sometimes a wound or some slight abrasion
gives the hæmolytic streptococcus access to the
deeper layers of the skin. It may then spread
along the surface, causing redness, swelling, and
much pain, more especially as it usually attacks
the skin of the face. This disease is known as *erysipelas*. The patient may generally expect to recover in the course of ten days or so, but if his resistance is low or the streptococcus very virulent, he
may become very gravely ill or even lose his life.
New-born infants are susceptible to the disease
and it is very fatal to them.

Other organs attacked are the ear, giving rise
to middle age disease, and, in rare cases, the
membranes of the brain, causing 'streptococcal
meningitis,' which may be said to have had an
invariably fatal termination. Other organs such
as the lung, the kidney, the bladder, the tonsils,
etc., may be affected. A variety of this streptococcus is also the cause of scarlet fever.

Domagk's announcement of a remedy for diseases of this class aroused interest, but not, as the
layman might expect, a wild enthusiasm. It is a
sobering experience to read the medical papers
and to compare the great number of new drugs
and treatments announced with the small proportion that are still in use five years later. A medical
man who tried every new discovery on his patients would have little chance to acquire the

technique of any or to observe their results. So prontosil was regarded with a scientific suspense of judgment until it had proved its worth. Even before Domagk's paper was published, prontosil had been tried out in various German clinical institutions and so some sixteen reliable and independent observers in Germany were able to confirm his work. Very soon other countries followed the German lead, and in France, Tréfouel, Nitti, and Bovet showed that the effect of prontosil has nothing to do with its being a dye, but that it broke up in the body, giving a much simpler subsance which had been known since 1908 under

AZO GROUP IN VIRTUE
OF WHICH PRONTOSIL IS A DYE

PRONTOSIL

PARA-AMINOBENZENESULPHONAMIDE
(SULPHANILAMIDE)

the chemical name of *para-aminobenzenesulpho-namide*. This colorless crystalline substance, they showed, had the same effect as the red dye prontosil. It was protected by nobody's patents, it was cheap to make, and it soon became very popular.

Most chemical firms sold their own brand and every one gave it a different name. The substance is now sold under thirty-three different names, producing a remarkable confusion in the literature. Doctors have often tried patients with, let us say, sulphanilamide, and having no great success, put them on to streptocide or colsulanyde, unaware that they were in fact exactly the same drug. Its official title is now sulphanilamide. The naming and nature of these drugs is quite a study in itself and will be discussed in Chapter VI. As a preliminary we may remember that prontosil is the original red dye; sulphanilamide the simplest of the group; sulphapyridine or M & B 693 the most active and widely applicable. The whole class of drugs are known as sulphonamides. But before we consider what the chemists have done with the group, let us first look at the early results which caused such general amazement.

The sulphonamide drugs won their spurs in the most valuable of work, saving the lives of mothers. One of the main causes of maternal mortality has always been puerperal fever, the infection of the genital tract of the mother with hæmolytic streptococci. In the period before 1870 when the connection between bacteria and disease was not understood, puerperal fever was the despair of the accoucheur. In hospital wards — on an average — one mother in thirty died of this diease, and sometimes the proportion rose to terrifying levels and the wards had to be closed. Yet in the patient's homes, however tumbledown and unsanitary, the disease was relatively uncommon. The work of Lister proved to the world what had been hinted by some earlier workers, including Semmelweiss, Oliver Wendell Holmes, and Florence Nightingale, namely that a potent cause of puerperal fever was the hand of the obstetrician, and in particular that of the medical student who came, unsterilized and often unwashed, from the dissecting-room or from cases of surgical sepsis or of erysipelas. Once the cause was discovered the mortality from puerperal fever fell and by 1935 was no more than one death per six hundred and fifty births. This still meant that every year a thousand mothers lost their lives from this cause, but it seemed impossible to decrease the incidence of the disease. A nurse might pick up virulent hæmolytic streptococci from a case of tonsillitis; children in the mother's family might harbor the germ in infected throats and ears; in many cases the mode of entry of this common bacterium could not be traced. There was no cure for the disease. Sera, such as are described in Chapter II, were available but the general opinion was that they had no favorable influence on the course of the disease. Nearly a quarter of those who were affected died; if the bacteria invaded the blood-stream the mortality rose to three-quarters.

Very soon after Domagk's paper appeared, Colebrook and Kenny decided to try the new remedy for cases of puerperal fever at Queen Charlotte's Maternity Hospital. Even the scrupulous precautions there observed failed to prevent occasional cases of puerperal fever. During the preceding five years 24 per cent, or very nearly a quarter of the cases, infected with hæmolytic streptococci, had died. The drug was tried on sixty-four cases in 1935 and 1936 and the death-rate among these was the astonishingly low figure of 4.7 per cent. Since that time the administration of one of the sulphonamide drugs has become the invariable treatment for puerperal fever. The present opinion is that the simplest of them, sulphanilamide itself, is the most effective, though any of the drugs (except *uleron*) may be used with effect. Recent papers indicate that the mortality of puerperal cases treated in this way may be as low as 1.4 per cent. The statistics given on p. 135 seem to indicate that, if the treatment is fully and systematically applied, we may hope to see a yearly saving of the lives of seven or eight hundred mothers. To these must be added the lives of the children these mothers may bear later in life; nor should we forget the effect of a mother's care on the children who would, but for sulphonamide drugs, have been left motherless. It had been hoped that the disease might be prevented by giving the drug as a routine measure to all women. This has not on the whole proved to be a success, though it remains an attractive possibility.

It was these results which made the treatment famous. Before we consider the other and perhaps even greater things which it has done we should first consider the results of the labors of the chemists.

CHAPTER VI

THE SULPHONAMIDE GROUP OF DRUGS

*The synthesis of new drugs—M and B 693—The
nomenclature of these drugs—List of names
and formulæ—Mode of administration—
Dangers.*

THE success of prontosil and paraminobenzenesulphonamide had the immediate result
of setting all the research departments of the other
fine-chemical firms to work. Prontosil was covered by Bayer's patents, so it remained their monopoly, but the latter drug had been known since
1908 and could not be patented. So almost all
the fine-chemical firms brought out their own
brand of paraminobenzenesulphonamide and put
it on the market under a different name. At the
same time many of them started research in order
to find something as good or better than either of
these drugs. It was quite evident that the 'busi-
ness-end' of both these drugs was the group of
atoms:

$$-N-C \underset{C=C}{\overset{C-C}{\diagup\!\!\!\diagdown}} C-SO_2-N\diagup$$

So hundreds of chemists set to work to synthesize substances with this group of atoms in their

molecule, and dozens of pathologists tried them
out on thousands of mice. Thus the chemists might
start from the simple compound sulphanilamide:

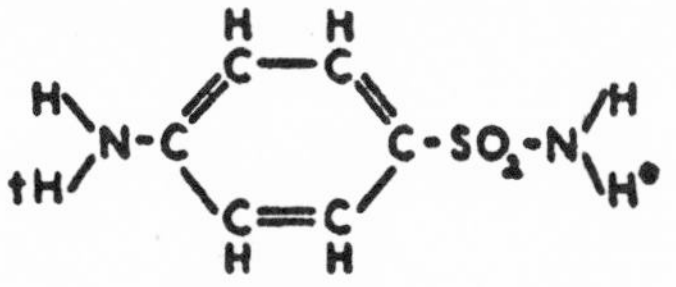

and try the effect of attacking other groups in the
place of hydrogen atoms marked †. Thus by putting a benzyl group

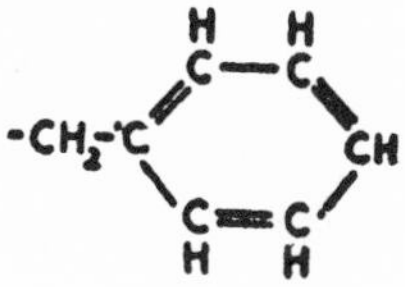

in the place of this hydrogen atom, the chemists of
Messrs. May and Baker obtained an active drug
with low toxicity (proseptasine). They then
naturally tried the effect of substituting a great
number of similar groups in the hope of finding
something still better. This hope, however, was
not rewarded. They then tried another line of
research, and various groups of atoms were put
in the place of the hydrogen atom marked *.
When the pyridyl group

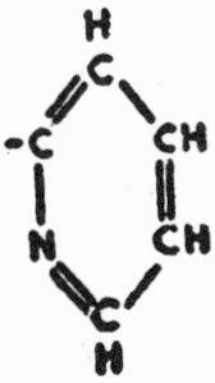

was attached at that point the highly active drug was produced which was given the laboratory number T 693 and was later introduced for clinical trial under the designation of M & B 693. Naturally this success led to the trial of a great number of groups containing what we call heterocyclic rings — rings of atoms containing both carbon atoms and other atoms. Most of these proved to be less useful than M & B 693. One, however, has been found to have a similar activity to the latter and also a greater activity against staphylococci. This has the group

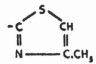

attached in place of the pyridyl of M & B 693, and is known as M & B 760a or sulphathiazole. Its activity against staphylococci is not spectacular; but work now in progress indicates that it may be extremely effective against certain other diseases, e.g. gonorrhœa and plague.

The result of this work to date has been that nine or ten new drugs of this type are being manufactured. It is not at all easy to say which of these is the 'best' in any particular conditions. The only sound way to compare them is for a hospital to divide its patients suffering from some disease into two batches and treat one of these with drug A and the other with drug B. This has not been done to any great extent as yet. The gen-

eral opinion at present is that sulphanilamide, rubiazol, red prontosil, and M & B 693 (sulphapyridine) are all about equally good for streptococcal
diseases; that M & B 693 alone is effective for
pneumonia; that M & B 693, sulphanilamide, and
uleron, are all useful in gonorrhœa. This really
boils down to the fact that M & B 693 is effective
for all conditions treatable in this way, but that
sulphanilamide, which is much cheaper, is an
adequate recourse in ailments other than those
caused by the pneumococcus. Rubiazol has the
advantage of being but slightly toxic. M & B 693
seems to be one of the safest of these drugs, and
would almost always be the drug of choice were
it not that it makes a great many patients feel
unpleasantly sick.

The table on pp. 140-175 gives a list of the drugs
in use, their makers, their chemical titles, formulæ, and trade-names.

The first thing that must strike the reader is
the remarkable confusion of the naming of these
drugs. The only logical name of each, from
which it could be identified is the chemical one:
unfortunately none of these names are concise and
that of prontosil-soluble is more like a speech than
a word. Consequently the drugs are usually known
by trade-names. There is no official body which
can settle the name of a new substance once and
for all. Certain medical societies occasionally try
to do so, but they cannot be sure that their suggestions will be adopted. Thus in America the
Council in Pharmacy and Chemistry of the Med-

ical Association chose the name sulphapyridine, the makers encourage the use of the name Dagenan, while in English medical journals it as often appears as M & B 693, or even simply 693. The name sulphanilamide is now usually adopted in medical literature, but in the earlier papers it is often described as sulphonamide-P, colsulanyde or prontosil album. Chemical journals commonly enforce a certain standard method of naming substances. It would be a great simplification if every new substance described in a communication or marketed for therapeutic purposes was given an official title by a committee of the central medical authority and if all chemical firms were to describe their products by this title with some addendum to show its origin. Pure chemicals are sold to research chemists under the same titles, no matter who is the vendor. If the latter believes his name or brand to be a recommendation he may add it; but he retains the universally accepted title. Thus he may sell his purest potassium permanganate as potassium permanganate Analar or potassium permanganate Judactan, but he never calls it Permangol or Condan or gives it any title which conceals its nature. To the scientific worker there seems a certain flavor of quackery about the fantastic multiplication of synonyms for the same drug.

It is interesting to compare the chemical formulæ of these drugs and to see that in all of them is found the single atom-pattern shown in heavier type. It is evidently this grouping which constitutes, so to speak, the wards of the key which fits the bacterium's lock. We have no idea why this should be so, nor do we understand how the rest of the atom-pattern modifies this power, as it undoubtedly does. Thus it is the pyridyl group

which distinguishes sulphapyridine (M & B 693), which attacks the pneumococcus, from the other drugs of the group which do not; and so presumably this pyridyl group in some way interlocks with something which is in the *pneumococcus* but not in *streptococcus pyogenes*. But we have no idea why the pyridyl group should affect the pneumococcus, and indeed the search for new drugs of this type is little more than trial and error: we have no idea of the possibilities of success. Thus, if a number of experts were asked whether they thought that a sulphonamide drug capable of affecting the tubercle bacillus could be discovered, they could do no more than say they did not know.

Most tantalizing is the realization that since ten years ago we had no idea that the sulphonamide group would affect bacteria, there may be half a dozen other groupings of atoms with the same or even much greater effect — and we have nothing to hint to us what groups they may be. If the researches on the way in which these drugs do their work (pp. 162-163) yield any result, we may be put in the position of being able to proceed rationally and not by mere trial and error. There is to-day more hope of this happy result than there was a year ago.

These sulphonamide drugs, unlike most of the earlier chemotherapeutic agents, are administered by mouth. This is an advantage in that it makes it possible for the patient to take medicine under the doctor's direction but in his absence; it is, however, a disadvantage where the patient is so gravely ill that he is unable to swallow. This is not uncommon with such diseases as cerebrospinal meningitis. The drugs work well if injected into a vein, but since the doses are large and many of these drugs require a great deal of water to dissolve them this is not always easy. Some very much more soluble products have recently been prepared to allow of this way of treatment.

Unlike most other synthetic drugs, they have to be taken in quite large quantities if they are to have any effect. Thus if sulphanilamide is the drug of choice, a gramme of it (equal in bulk to about three aspirin tablets) is given at a time. The body gets rid of the drug again pretty quickly, so a dose is usually given every four hours — even if the patient has to be wakened in the night to take it. This treatment is kept up for from five to ten days so that the patient may take in all 30 to 60 grammes (1 to 2 oz.) of the drugs. It is of no use at all to swallow an occasional tablet; even a course of the drug lasting two or three days may leave a few living bacteria behind which will then multiply anew and reproduce the disease. This heavy dosing is one reason why these drugs should not be sold to the patient who wants to doctor himself without medical advice. If he takes only a few tablets no good result occurs, and if he takes the full dosage he is subjecting himself to a process which requires to be watched by a doctor, for overdoses of these drugs may have unpleasant effects. In the first place, even the ordinary medicinal doses commonly make the patient feel ill and look ill, a result which may be alarming but is generally quite harmless and temporary. The patient and, worse still, his relatives are apt to be frightened when, as is quite common, he assumes a peculiar leaden color. This effect is due to an alteration in a part of the red blood pigment; in some cases this is due to the combination of sulphur compounds with the blood, and so sulphur-containing foods such as eggs and onions have to be avoided, and also certain purgatives, such as Epsom salts. A curious "drug-fever" also sometimes crops up, but does not seem to be very serious.

But there is one complication which must be looked on as the real drawback of these drugs. Occasionally they act as poisons to the cells in the bone-marrow which have the essential task of producing white blood cells, and bring about a condition which may lead to death within a few days. About fifty deaths have been recorded: it is hard to conjecture what proportion this is of the patients treated, but as a guess it would seem to be less than one in a thousand. The drugs would then seem to be only about as dangerous as a general anæsthetic. Agranulocytosis, as the effect is termed, is becoming a rarer complication now that the danger is known, and an examination of the patient's blood is commonly made a routine, for by examining and counting the blood cells the doctor can detect any deficiency and stop the administration of the drug. A mortality of even one in a thousand is obviously no reason to eschew these drugs in ailments with a high mortality such as puerperal fever or pneumonia, for where the chance of death is being lowered from one in four to one in twelve, the additional chance of one in a thousand due to possible agranulocytosis is negligible. On the other hand this small chance of fatality inclines the cautious practitioner to avoid the use of these drugs in diseases which have no direct mortality, such as the common cold. It seems probable indeed that colds are cut short after some two days by these drugs, but since their use is mildly unpleasant and, as we have seen, not entirely free from danger, we must not expect them to free us from this curse.

CHAPTER VII

SULPHONAMIDES AND STREPTOCOCCUS PYOGENES

Streptococci—Puerperal fever—Saving of life— Cellulitis — Blood-poisoning — War wounds — Erysipelas — Chronic infections — Endocarditis.

THE organism which is responsible for most septic wounds and blood-poisoning, for puerperal fever, erysipelas, etc., is *streptococcus pyogenes,* which is commonly called the β-hæmolytic streptococcus. There are probably over thirty distinguishable types of *streptococcus pyogenes,* and those strains classed as group A are responsible for about 90 per cent of human streptococcal infections. This group A is sensitive to sulphonamide drugs. Concerning the rare infections with other types of streptococci less is known, but it seems that many of them are resistant to sulphonamide drugs. It cannot be said that we yet know which of these drugs is the most active against streptococci, but sulphanilamide itself has been most widely used. Its chemical simplicity and the fact that it is not patented make it less expensive than the others, and so, in absence of any definite contra-indication, it tends to be most widely used.

The most spectacular results have been obtained in puerperal fever. Colebrook and Kenny's results have already been mentioned (p. 122), and other workers have found the same remarkable drop in mortality. Thus Foulis and Barr in 1937 reported twenty-two cases with only one death; for the five preceding years the mortality-rate of their puerperal fever cases had been 17.4 per cent, while this series shows only 1.4 per cent. Another series showed only two deaths in thirty-nine cases, some of which were extremely severe. The mortality of puerperal fever is a very variable one, but these rates are so far below anything previously known that it is impossible to attribute the low mortality to a diminution in the virulence of the bacteria.

The obstetrician rightly regards the prevention of puerperal fever as being a duty quite as imperative as its cure. The attempt to prevent the infection by administering the drug to lying-in women has been tried. Some positive and some negative results have been obtained, but there seems to be an opinion that where there is considered to be a special risk of infection, e.g. when there is operative interference, the drug should be employed.

The number of published results is not sufficient to give a clear idea of the number of lives such treatment might save, but the series which have been recorded seems to indicate that at least three-quarters of the deaths from puerperal fever will be prevented. The Registrar General's

Report gives the following figures for the number of deaths from this cause per 100,000 births:

	1930	1931	1932	1933	1934	1935	1936*	1937	1938
Deaths from sepsis per 100,000 births	184	159	155	175	195	161	134	94	86

If we take the average mortality before the treatment as 171 per 100,000 births and assume that sulphonamide treatment can save three-quarters, the death-rate from this cause should come down to 43 per 100,000, but this is not likely to be realized, for it would indicate that every mother would be receiving the care and observation which would be hers in a great hospital. In England and Wales in 1938 there were 645,933 births, and the reduction of mortality from the 171 average of 1930-1935 to the 1938 figure of 86 means that 549 mothers were saved— in all probability as a direct result of the use of this drug, and there is, it would seem, a good chance of saving perhaps two or three hundred more each year. Moreover, it is not in England and Wales alone that such lives are being saved. We may reflect on, if we cannot assess, the number of those being rescued from death in Europe and America with a population nearly twenty times that of England and Wales.

It is not only the injuries of childbirth which

*Sulphonamide Treatment introduced.

can become infected with *streptococcus pyogenes*. It is, in fact, to be found in the majority of infected wounds. The bacterium varies greatly in the violence of its invasion. Sometimes, indeed usually, it remains localized in the wound; patients then as a rule exhibit some degree of fever and illness, but are likely to recover. Sometimes it invades the tissues and even the blood-stream, giving rise to a very grave state of affairs. In peace-time cases of this type are not very common and few have been reported, yet one of the first of them had in it a quality of appropriateness which usually belongs rather to fiction than fact.

While prontosil was still at the experimental stage under the direction of Domagk, his own daughter happened to thrust a needle into her hand, and by ill-chance to introduce with it virulent streptococci. The bacteria multiplied, invaded the surrounding tissues, and gave rise to a rapidly spreading cellulitis with its usual inflammation, pain, and illness. Surgical treatment —the free opening up of the infected area, etc. —was employed, but with no avail. She became desperately ill and, as a last resort, when she was sinking fast, the new and hardly tried-out drug was administered. The results were dramatic. She rallied and made a complete recovery. Rarely is it that a research worker's reward is so rapid and direct.

Such cases have since then been multiplied many times. As early as 1935, an operation wound

in a surgeon's finger, which was showing signs
of blood-poisoning, was treated by administering
prontosil and his life saved. There is no doubt
that many of the community's most valuable
lives have been saved and will be saved in this
way.

It was shown in the last war that the usual
cause of infection in war wounds was *streptococcus pyogenes,* the source of which was probably the noses, throats, and hands of the many
people who came in contact with the patient before he reached hospital. The total number of
deaths, from injuries as distinguished from sickness, resulting from the war of 1914-1918 has
been estimated as seven and a quarter millions.
It appears that about three-quarters of these
deaths took place on the battlefield and about
one-quarter in hospital. The chief cause of death
in hospital was the activities of *streptococcus
pyogenes,* and it would seem reasonable to ascribe
at least a million deaths to this bacterium. If, as
seems likely, the rate of diminution of mortality
proves to be the same for wound-infections as
for puerperal sepsis, we may conclude that sulphanilamide or M & B 693 could have saved
seven hundred and fifty thousand men. To-day
the War Office has prescribed that sulphanilamide shall be administered to all wounded men;
it is reported (June, 1940) that the good condition of the wounds of men so treated is in striking
contrast to that of similar wounds seen in the
war 1914-18.

In erysipelas — streptococcal infection of the skin — the new drugs work like a charm. In nearly 90 per cent of cases infection ceases to spread within twenty-four hours and recovery quickly completes itself. In one set of three hundred and twelve cases, those treated with prontosil showed one death in forty, while those treated according to the most approved of former methods showed one death in fifteen. Moreover, the time needed for the recovery of prontosil-treated cases was far shorter and the consequent pain and temporary disablement far less. In infants under two years old erysipelas has in the past been a very deadly disease from which only one child in four or five recovered: to-day the picture is wholly changed and it seems that only one child in eight or ten need die from this disease.

The infection of the brain by streptococci — *Streptococcal meningitis* — is a particular field of triumph for the new drugs. It is a rare disease, which occasionally follows erysipelas of the head or an infected middle ear, and it was almost uniformly fatal. Thus in one series of twenty-one cases only one recovered: when the new drugs were tried, four out of the next seven cases recovered: in another series of thirty-nine cases, thirty-two recovered!

It is a curious fact that these drugs are most effective in the most desperate cases, where the bacteria are, so to speak, attacking in open country. Where the bacteria are entrenched in some septic organ sulphonamide drugs are less certain in their effect. Thus acute tonsillitis is cured in a spectacular fashion, but it is by no means so easy to destroy the bacteria in chronically septic tonsils, discharging ears, septic mastoids, infected bladders or kidneys. In such cases the action of the drugs is uncertain. Sometimes they work extremely well and completely eradicate the disease; sometimes they improve it greatly, but leave a few bacteria still capable of giving trouble; sometimes they have no effect whatever. Yet in all these conditions, the practitioner has received a most valuable aid, for this uncertainty of action is shared by most drugs, and appears unsatisfactory only by contrast with the remarkable effect of sulphonamide drugs on the acute cases we have mentioned.

While the group A *streptococcus pyogenes* is the cause of most of our more serious streptococcal infections, there is one very serious disease which results from infection of the interior of the heart with another type of streptococcus, *streptococcus viridans*. This disease, known as malignant endocarditis, seems to occur as the result of some other acute infection. Recovery takes place in only 2 or 3 per cent of the cases, and the disease causes some two thousand five hundred deaths each year in England and Wales. The bacteria lodge in what are called 'vegetations,' masses of fibrin (blood-clot) that collect on the valves of the heart. Portions of these often break away and lodge in other organs, causing further troubles. Sulphapyridine (M & B 693) is quite active against the *streptococcus viridans,* but although it seems to influence these cases favorably for a time, it does not bring about recovery. Sulphonamide drugs seem to do their work only in presence of blood-serum (p. 161), but within these 'vegetations' there is little blood supply, and some at least of the bacteria survive.

CHAPTER VIII

PNEUMONIA AND M & B 693

The pneumococcus — Pneumonia — Mortality-rate
of pneumonia — M and B 693 — Statistics
of treatment — Broncho-pneumonia — Pneu-
mococcal meningitis — American attitude

THE word *pneumonia* does not describe a
single disease, but means simply an inflammation of the lung-substance. This inflammation
is due to bacteria growing in the lung and these
can be of many different types. Thus *streptococcus pyogenes* can cause pneumonia, and such cases
can be treated by any sulphonamide drug. However, the disease which the man in the street calls
pneumonia is what the doctors call *acute lobar
pneumonia.*

The infecting bacterium in such cases is the
streptococcus pneumoniæ which is usually re-
ferred to as the *pneumococcus.* It is one of the
bacteria of which many strains exist, and there
are some thirty-four strains of it which can be
distinguished by the way they react to antisera.
Some very interesting work has been done on
these. It appears that the bacteria consist of two
main portions — first, an outer capsule made of

a material resembling the vegetable gums which is of different constitution in each of the thirty-four strains, and inside this the protoplasm of the bacterium itself which is the same in all the strains. The bacteria of different strains are, in fact, the same creatures in different skins. There does not seem to be any evidence that any one strain is more resistant to chemotherapy than any other, which gives this treatment a considerable advantage over serum-therapy to which each behaves differently.

The *streptococcus pneumoniæ* seems to be a usual inhabitant of our noses and throats, but not of our air-ways (bronchi) or lungs. No doubt it must continually find its way from our noses to our lungs, but in the normal course of events it is effectively removed (p. 51). But now and again some incident renders the removal mechanism ineffective, or lowers the resistance of the tissues to infection. This incident may be a lowering of the temperature of the body or an invasion of the lung by some other organism, such as the influenza virus. The pneumococcus then colonizes some part of one or both lungs. The result is an acute inflammation of the tiny—almost microscopic—air-cells where the blood circulating in the lung-tissue receives from the air its load of vitally necessary oxygen. The inflamed blood-vessels pour out into these cells a liquid which coagulates to a solid mass, blocking up the air-spaces completely. Generally only a part of one lung is affected, so the patient does not die from lack of air. He is, however, gravely ill from absorption of the bacterial toxins. In favorable cases the matter which blocks up the air-cells is liquefied and absorbed, so that the lung recovers completely. In unfavorable cases the bacteria invade the blood and the patient may die from infection of the heart or often of the brain.

The disease is a common one and in England and Wales some fifty or sixty thousand cases occur every year. Of these somewhere between a fifth and a quarter have a fatal termination and, consequently, the mortality from the disease can be put at some twelve thousand deaths a year. In North America both the number of cases and the mortality-rate are higher than in England and Wales.

The treatment of pneumonia for a long time consisted in little else but good nursing, that is to say, the providing of conditions in which the body can best mobilize and apply its defense-mechanisms. In recent years, vaccines have been employed, but their results, though useful, have not been very impressive, chiefly because there are some thirty strains of pneumococci, and sera made from one strain did not fully protect against the others. The mortality-rate of the disease in temperate countries rarely fell below 20 per cent, and was usually higher. It is a disease which has victims of all ages, but which is much more fatal to the old than to the young. Roughly speaking, half of those above the age of fifty, who contracted pneumonia, died of it, while of those below the age of fifty, only about one in seven failed to recover; while below the age of twenty, there is only about one fatal case in twenty-five.

Since pneumonia is so common and so fatal a disease, any advance in its treatment means a notable saving of lives. A very great discovery, then, was made when Dr. A. J. Ewins and Mr. M. A. Phillips, in the research laboratories of Messrs. May and Baker, Ltd., produced a sulphonamide drug which, unlikely any other member of the group, had a powerful effect upon the pneumococcus. The discovery was not a chance one, for a great number of drugs of the sulphanilamide group had been synthesized in the hope of finding one which had such activity. This drug is 2-sulphanilyl-amidopyridine, which has attained fame as M & B 693 and is now known under that name or the official title of sulphapyridine. Its formula, given below, shows us that it is practically sulphanilamide with the pyridyl group

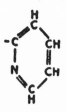

hitched on to the sulphanilamide molecule

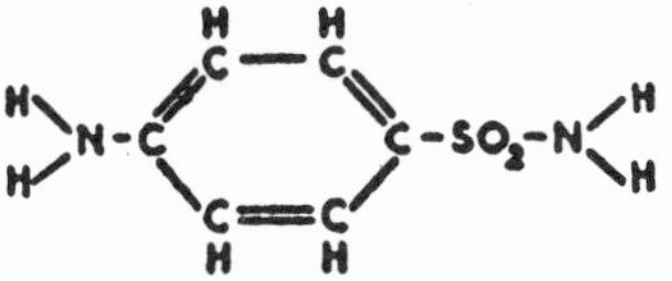

SULPHANILAMIDE

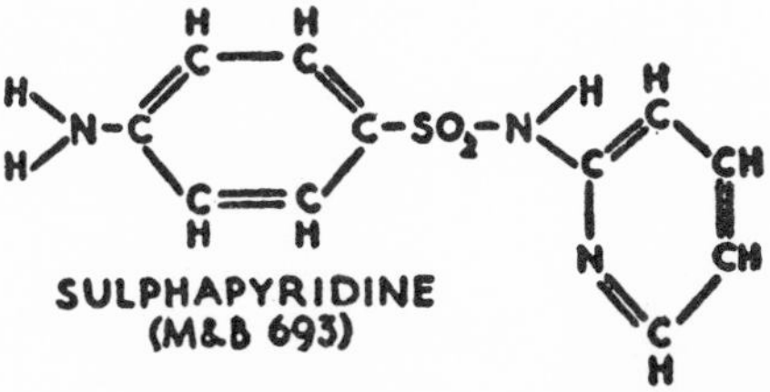

SULPHAPYRIDINE (M&B 693)

PYRIDYL GROUP

It is not the only drug in the series which attacks the pneumococcus, but it is the one which has the best 'therapeutic ratio' — that is to say, is most poisonous to the bacteria and least poisonous to the patient. It is a white and slightly bitter powder which dissolves only to a slight extent in water. A soluble modification is also now available.

The discoverer of the activity of the drug was Dr. L. E. H. Whitby who examined a large number of the new drugs which Messrs. May and Baker's chemists had synthesized. The work was, of course, complicated by the fact that there are a large number of 'strains' or 'types' of the pneumococcus. Mice were inoculated with bacteria of each type: some were dosed with M & B 693 and some were left untreated. The results were spectacular. In one series of experiments the mice received 50,000 Type I pneumococci apiece. The sixty controls, who were untreated, were dead within an average of seventeen hours: while of the seventy-two mice which received the same number of bacteria and also a dose of 30 or 40 milligrams of the new drug, one and all survived. The other types of pneumococcus were also tested and the drug was found to be efficacious against them though not so much so as against Type I. Whitby, moreover, showed that M & B 693 was equal to or better than sulphanilamide in curing streptococcal diseases.

Whitby's results were very impressive, and in the same year the drug was tried out on human patients with remarkable success by Drs. Evans and Gaisford at the Dudley Road Hospital, Birmingham. First it was ascertained that healthy human beings could take large doses with impunity. Then, in March, 1938, the lobar pneumonia patients entering the hospital were divided into two groups, one of which received M & B 693, while the other was treated by the best methods previously known. The result was very much better than anything which could have been expected. Eight of the hundred patients treated with M & B 693 died, as against twenty-seven of the hundred patients who constituted the control group. Not only did more of the treated patients recover, but they also suffered much less severely and recovered in a shorter time than the controls.

Further controlled tests were felt to be unnecessary and, indeed, unjustifiable, and, since

July 1938, M & B 693 has been the standard treatment for pneumonia.

Since that time many more figures have become available, and the number of patients reported on amount to three thousand or so. The figures make it clear that the mortality of pneumonia patients treated with M & B 693 is from 1/8 to 1/3 of the mortality of untreated patients. Thus in England the mortality of patients treated in this way is 5 to 8 per cent, whereas without the drug it is 20 to 27 per cent. Generally speaking, in warmer countries the usual mortality is lower and in colder countries higher than the above figures. Thus in a series reported from Kenya, only 16 per cent of the controls died, and only 2 per cent of those receiving the drug.

If we adopt the figures of 20 per cent mortality-rate without the drug and 5.3 per cent with it, resulting from the study of about 1600 cases at the Dudley Road Hospital, it would seem that if the treatment were applied to every lobar pneumonia case, about 7500 lives a year would be saved in this country alone — and no doubt a great proportion of these are being saved already. What are 7500 lives worth in cash? I do not know, but I should be prepared to pay a very high figure for my own. No public money was expended on this discovery; yet if the nation had spent a million on it, should we call it dear at the price?

The rate at which discoveries such as this are made depends precisely on the time spent on trying to make them, which depends equally precisely on the money available for research. The great commercial firms have done exceedingly fine work in this matter, but the quantity of research they can do must necessarily depend on the profits they earn, for this, after all, is the sole source of their funds. We can accelerate the work to exactly the extent we choose by putting our hands in our pockets to pay for such work to be done in public institutions.

To return to our pneumonia treatment. Contrary to general expectation and to the indications of the first experiments on mice, the new drug has proved equally successful for infections with any of the strains of pneumococcus encountered. It is effective both for young and old. Thus in one long series of cases it was found that, of those under fifty, one in seventy die instead of one in seven: of those over fifty, two in nine die, instead of one in two.

There is another type of pneumonia known as bronchopneumonia in which the wider air-tubes of the lungs are infected with bacteria. These are usually a mixed bag drawn from any or all of the types which commonly infest the throat. Naturally, M & B 693 is not so effective in bronchopneumonia because many of the bacteria belong to species which are unharmed by it. Yet it appears that the mortality of this disease, which causes some seventeen thousand deaths each year in this country, can be reduced at least to half or a third of its normal value, so opening up the possibility of saving some eight thousand lives each year.

Like the streptococcus — though not to the same extent — the pneumococcus can infect several parts of the body. Its usual habitat is the lung, but it can infect the membranes of the brain, to which it presumably finds it way *via* the nose, in which pneumococci are usually to be found. This results in a disease termed *pneumococcal meningitis* which had the unhappy reputation of causing 100 per cent mortality. It is not very easily distinguished from the other forms of meningitis, but this is not important in practice, for M & B 693 is very effective in nearly all of these. The number of cases in which M & B 693 has been employed is not enough to establish any mortality figure, but it would seem that the patient has now a good expectation of recovery (*c.* 50%) from this disease which was formerly invariably fatal.

In this country, at any rate, almost unqualified approval has been accorded to this new treatment for pneumonia. Undoubtedly there are cases which prove resistant to the drug, but the evidence available has convinced our medical men that treatment with M & B 693 is a vast improvement on treatment with sera.

In America a less warm welcome was given to the new therapy. First of all a very unfortunate happening prejudiced the American public against the sulphonamide drugs. A firm at Tulsa, Oklahoma, in 1937 put on the market a preparation of sulphanilamide dissolved in a mixture of 72 per cent diethyleneglycol and water. The man-

ufacturers appear to have concluded that diethyleneglycol — which is a chemical not unlike
glycerine—was a harmless inert substance, whereas it appears to be very dangerous. Their preparation caused a shocking series of deaths, which
were at first attributed to the sulphanilamide.
European experience, of course, entirely exoner-
ates the latter drug, and the deaths were pretty
certainly due to the diethyleneglycol. None the
less it was not a good start for the sulphanilamide
drugs. However, they have since largely recovered from the set-back and are widely in use.

When the English results for pneumonia treatment were first announced, some of the American
medical journals considered that the new treatment was being adopted on the basis of too little
evidence — too short a series of cases. The Amer-
icans had studied the statistics of serum treatment
of pneumonia with very great exactness and perhaps our series of a hundred or two cases looked
a little slender. There are now, however, numerous reports of the use of this treatment in the
U. S. A. We hear of the mortality from pneumonia in a great American hospital being cut by
two-thirds, and no doubt the new treatment will
completely establish itself within a year or so —
unless something even better takes its place.

CHAPTER IX

FURTHER TRIUMPHS

*Meningitis — Cerebrospinal meningitis — Spectacular results from Sudan — Gonorrhœa — Its dangers — Treatment with **sulphanila-**mide or M & B 693 — Reasons against self-treatment — Effect of sulphonamides on Bacterium coli and staphylococci — Effect on plague — Veterinary uses — **Limitations** of the treatment — Mode of action.*

THE term *meningitis* simply means an inflammation of the meninges, or lining membrane of the brain and spinal cord. This inflammation, which is always extremely dangerous, can be caused by infection with any of quite a number of species of bacteria. The β-hæmolytic streptococcus or the pneumococcus may cause it, with results which were almost invariably fatal before the introduction of sulphonamides. The tubercle bacillus may also cause it and — since no chemotherapeutic agent attacks this formidable man-slayer — death is almost always the result.

There is a form of meningitis much commoner than these, caused by a bacterium, the meningococcus, or *Neisseria meningitidis,* which does not generally infect other parts of the body. The mortality-rate of 40 per cent is low, one of 70 per cent normal, and 90 per cent not uncommon.

Worst of all it is an epidemic disease, conveyed, it is supposed, in the noses and throats of *carriers,* persons who harbor the bacterium but do not suffer from the disease. It seems to be conveyed by droplets of sputum and so may have terrible effects where there is over-crowding and little ventilation. Thus it caused serious epidemics in the war of 1914-1918, where troops were closely herded together in barracks or huts. Over four thousand cases with nearly two thousand deaths occurred, a mortality-rate of 40 per cent. In the present war the mortality-rate has been but 8 per cent, a result entirely attributable to the new treatment.

During the last decade cerebrospinal meningitis has caused, each year, between one thousand five hundred and three thousand five hundred deaths. The only treatment of any avail was a serum. This had its value, but even with serum treatment the mortality remained very high. In England (1931-1938) untreated cases had a 60 to 70 per cent mortality; in those treated with serum the mortality was about 37 per cent. In 1936 Buttle tested the effect of sulphanilamide on mice infected with meningococci and demonstrated that it would both protect them against infection and also cure the disease. A number of workers in 1937 and 1938 tried sulphanilamide with success, and in the same year Dr. Hobson and Mr. McQuaide at the Radcliffe Infirmary, Oxford, used

M & B 693 in treating six cases, all of which recovered.   Later Banks used the drug in seventy-
two cases and had only one death in the series —
a mortality of only 1.4 per cent.

A very interesting series of cases hails from the
Sudan.   There has been in past years a considerable mortality from this disease in the Anglo-
Egyptian Sudan, and Usher Somers, and also
Bryant and Fairman, carried out there a research
much more extensive than any which had been
possible in this country.   In the years 1934-1938
there were 21,599 cases in the Sudan and 14,816
died, giving a mortality-rate of 68 per cent — two
deaths in three.   Soon after the new drugs became
available in the Sudan, an outbreak of meningitis
recurred.   It was evidently a severe one, for thirty-
three patients had died out of forty-one attacked.   The disease was combated by injection of
M & B 693.   The drug could not be given in the
usual fashion, for it is not possible to administer
drugs by mouth to a powerful African deprived
of his reason by meningitis; the drug was, therefore, administered by injection.   Its success was
spectacular.   One medical officer had 129 recov-
eris out of 143 cases — another had 181 recoveries out of 189.   A death-rate of 69 per cent, or
worse, had been converted into one of 5 to 10 per
cent.

The drugs gained a testimonial from an unex-
pected source.   The local medicine-men, who normally drive a very lucrative trade, actually advised

those who came to them to go to the white doctors, who alone seemed to be able to influence this dread disease.

Closely allied to the *Neisseria meningitidis,* which causes cerebrospinal meningitis, is the *Neisseria gonorrhœa,* or gonococcus, which causes the venereal disease of gonorrhœa. The other important disease of this character — syphilis — has been enormously diminished both in quantity and severity by Ehrlich's arsenical drugs, discussed on pp. 91-92. Gonorrhœa, on the other hand, remained till 1937 a rather intractable infection. Since the disease has no immediate mortality, it has in the past been regarded as no very serious matter — unpleasant enough for the victim, but since he brought his trouble on himself, a matter for hilarity among his friends. But we have gradually come to realize that this ailment is not quite so funny. It involved its victims in a treatment lasting some three months; and, if he neglected this treatment, he might find himself the victim of infection of the joints, producing the effect of a most intractable and severe arthritis. But if this were all he might well regard the victim with little sympathy; for the exercise of continence, or common sense, enables the disease to be avoided. The true significance of the disease is not the effect on the patient but on his family. Gonorrhœa is, of course, highly contagious and so a considerable proportion of its victims are the innocent marriage partners of unfaithful spouses. This would be bad enough, but there is worse. The human eye is an ideal breeding-ground for these bacteria, and the intense inflammation they set up can destroy its sight in a few hours. A mother may be infected with the disease. She may believe herself cured or, if she is ignorant and accustomed to ill-health, she may never know nor even inquire what is the matter with her. When her baby is born, its eyes become infected with the germs and blindness results. There are some five thousand cases a year of this infection of the eyes of the new-born. Most of these do not now lead to blindness, for it is now the rule that new-born babies' eyes shall be disinfected as a routine, but none the less it is estimated that a quarter of the blind children in the country — some four thousand five hundred — are blind from this cause, and that another third are blind as the result of hereditary syphilis. Blindness has been steadily decreasing — and the progress of treatment by chemotherapy and of the health education which alone causes people to seek treatment and persevere with it will further diminish this heavy scourge.

The discovery that the sulphonamide drugs were able to kill the gonococcus was made in 1937. At first the colored prontosils were tried — then sulphanilamide. At this stage there was some dispute as to the degree of efficacy of these drugs. The decisive step was the discovery that the drug M & B 693 (sulphapyridine) had an exceptionally strong influence upon the gonococcus. The drug was tried out in 1938 and proved

to be much more efficacious than any of the others.
In ordinary uncomplicated cases the effect is
dramatic.   The very unpleasant symptoms and
outward signs of the disease vanish in a dramatic
fashion and in a majority of cases a course of the
drug lasting four or five days makes the patient
appear and feel perfectly well.   Such a success,
to quote one authority, 'sounded like a fairy story
to venerologists,' and very soon became known
even to the general public.   In many countries a
serious problem was created by sufferers from the
disease buying the tablets at the chemist's and
treating themselves.   There is always a danger with
venereal diseases, for some patients are loath to
acknowledge their condition even to their own
doctor.

Why should they not treat themselves?   There
are two excellent reasons.   The first is that the
patient has no means of telling when he is free from
the gonococcus and therefore from infectiveness.
The fact of feeling well and the disappearance of
all visible symptoms does not imply the absence
of the infecting bacteria.   There are two tests
which will indicate whether the disease is in fact
cured.   These are the microscope and the patient's
marriage partner.   Professional treatment employs
the first and self-treatment the second.   The only
way to be sure of not spreading the infection is a
bacterial examination which shows the gonococcus to be absent — or preferably several such ex-
aminations.

A second reason against self-treatment is the

occasional failure of the drug to do its work. Sulphonamide drugs are recognized as the first and
normal recourse, but the medical profession recog-
nizes that a proportion of patients, perhaps 10 to
20 per cent, show no improvement. Sometimes
these cases can be cured by the use of a different
sulphonamide drug; thus those which are not affected by sulphanilamide may be cured by uleron.
In addition to these wholly resistant cases, there
is a small number which relapse after a few weeks
or months — and these relapsed cases are often
resistant to the drug and must be cured by the
old and slower methods.

There are two enormous advantages of the new
method over the older ones. First, it makes patients much more ready to seek treatment. The
general public is rather vague in its ideas about
such things, but its bad conscience makes it believe that the ordinary treatment is at least unpleasant. The idea may be quite a false one, but its
effect is not the less. When the venereal public
understands that all it will be asked to endure will
be the taking of some tablets and, as a result,
suffering no worse inconvenience than feeling a bit
off color, it will no longer hesitate to seek treatment. Secondly, it appears that M & B 693 renders 90 per cent of male cases non-infectious in
the first week of treatment, whereas the old treatment left them infectious for two or three months.
Clearly, then, the number of potential sources of
infection will be greatly diminished and it is said
that the incidence of the disease is already mark-

edly on the wane. Patients are, moreover, disabled
for a much less period. Soldiers, who by reason of
their vigorous but technically celibate life are pecu-
liarly exposed to such diseases, were formerly
disabled from full duty for two or three months
— to-day, the period is about three weeks.

We are now nearing the end of our list of the
successes of sulphonamide treatment and coming
to those applications of it whose value stands as
yet in doubt.

It seems clear that the drug is a powerful agent
for destroying *Bacillus coli,* the usually harmless
inhabitant of our large intestines. This bacterium
is not killed by sulphonamide drugs as long as it
remains in this site, nor is there any particular
reason to wish to kill it. *Bacillus coli,* and other
intestinal bacteria, are, however, very apt to enter
the urinary system from without, and to cause
persistent infections of the kidneys and bladder,
from which they are not easily expelled. It has
been found that *B. coli* is very readily removed
from the urinary system by sulphanilamide, which
is normally excreted in the urine. Other intestinal
flora, are, however, not so easily killed in this way;
for these another synthetic drug, mandelic acid,
is preferred.

Finally these drugs are very valuable in the
cure of two venereal diseases which are not very
common in this country, though more so in the
tropics, namely, chancroid and lymphogranuloma
inguinale. Besides, these diseases which are certainly benefited by sulphonamides there are a

great number about which authorities are not agreed. The staphylococcal infections are a good example. Staphylococci are mostly skin-dwellers and cause boils, pimples, carbuncles, and so forth; they may, however, cause serious abscesses — whitlows — or even blood-poisoning. The published results seem to indicate that the sulphonamide drugs are of some value, though by no means a certain cure. The fact that they have some influence gives us good hope that a chemotherapeutic remedy for staphylococci may be found: much work is being done on this point, and the new drug mentioned on p. 126 is an indication of possible success.

The drugs have been tried on patients suffering from many other diseases. Favorable results have been found in the treatment of plague, but only a very few cases have been studied. Experiments on animals indicate that M & B 693 is active against *Pasteurella pestis,* the plague bacterium. Carman in 1938 found that three out of six patients treated with the drugs recovered while nine controls died. This is very encouraging, but the numbers are too small for anything approaching proof. Some success has also been had with the deadly gas-gangrene which carried off so many of the wounded in the war of 1914-1918.

Finally there would be a certain justice in the use of these drugs for treatment of the diseases of animals, for the lives of many animals have been necessarily sacrificed in the testing of their efficacy. There is no reason why these drugs should be less effective in the treatment of animal infections than in human. In certain types of illness there has indeed been very good success. Pigs are very susceptible to infection with the bacterium which we call *Hæmophilus influenzæ suis*. This causes forms of arthritis and also of pneumonia. Soluseptasine and M & B 693 have both proved to be successful in abolishing the mortality from this cause.

Other forms of animal pneumonia seem, according to preliminary results, to show promise of success. The drugs do not, however, seem to influence many of the worst animal diseases, e.g. foot-and-mouth disease and canine distemper, for these are virus-diseases, which, as a class, are not amenable to the known types of chemotherapy.

In recounting the many spectacular successes of chemotherapy, we must not forget its present limitations. There is still a long list of bacterial diseases which are not influenced by any drug. Tuberculosis, typhoid, paratyphoid, cholera, bacillary dysentery, whooping-cough, are unaffected by these drugs. But we do not know of any respect in which the bacteria which cause these diseases are essentially unlike those which are influenced by sulphonamides; so there is a reasonable hope that research may lead to remedies for some or all of these.

With the virus diseases, ultimate success is less probable, though by no means to be despaired of. It seems that one or two of the larger types of

virus particles are influenced by drugs. Lymphogranuloma inguinale mentioned above is a virus
disease; trachoma, a very serious and contagious
infection of the eyes, is reported to be very greatly
improved. But the main body of virus diseases is
uninfluenced. Smallpox, measles, infantile paralysis, colds, influenza, foot-and-mouth-disease, canine distemper, and so on, are not checked by any
drug. In some instances, however, the gravamen
of a virus disease lies in an invasion by bacteria
of the tissues previously weakened by the virus.
In this case, sulphonamide drugs may be of value.
Thus though they do not arrest the course of
smallpox they may prevent infection of the pustules by bacteria — so diminishing both illness
and scarring.

It may be that we have not yet found the right
drug to influence virus diseases. The body's defense mechanism can certainly destroy these
minutest of living particles, so it would seem theoretically possible to kill them by means of drugs.
But generally speaking the simpler and minuter
the parasite the harder it is to kill, for there are
in the simpler creatures fewer stages in the life-
process to be interfered with. If the simplest viruses consist of particles whose sole functions are to
assimilate ready-digested food material from the
cell-contents of its host, and to reproduce its kind,
there are only these two processes with which
drugs can interfere, in place of the hundreds of
which we may suppose to occur in a creature as
complicated as a trypanosome.

The search for other types of chemotherapeutic drug would be made much easier if we knew how these drugs acted on bacteria. The original idea of Ehrlich that they combined with the bacteria, as a dye does with wool, seems to be quite wrong.

In the first place the drugs are much less effective in killing bacteria outside the body than inside it; they are, in fact, rather poor disinfectants. The drugs and human blood-serum together are much more effective destroyers of bacteria than the drugs alone.

One view of the action of the drugs is that they destroy or prevent the formation of the protective capsules which usually surround the bacteria. There seems to be good evidence for this view, but even if it is correct, it is not very helpful since we do not know why there should be any affinity between the sulphonamide group of atoms and the capsules of the bacteria. Others have thought that the drugs combine with the toxins produced by the bacteria and neutralize their action, but the experimental evidence seems to be against this. A third theory is that the serum and sulphanilamide together form a substance which causes the white cells of the blood to be more active in attacking the bacteria. This view is not, however, generally accepted. It is curious that the drugs are intensely active against bacteria in their virulent phase when they are rapidly multiplying but have little or no effect when they are in the avirulent or 'rough' stage. Possibly the most favored view at the moment is that the drugs — presumably with the aid of something contained in blood-serum—destroy some substance in the bacterium, probably one of the enzymes, which are essential to its nutrition and growth.

These researches have not yet given any answer to the question: Why do sulphonamide drugs, rather than any other type, kill certain bacteria?   Consequently our search for other groups of chemotherapeutic drugs must still proceed by the laborious method of trial and error, and while this is the case our most urgent need is for a large volume of such work to be done — for many new drugs to be synthesized and tested.   The carrying out of such work does not require genius, but the more readily obtainable services of a large number of skilled organic chemists and bacteriologists. If we wish it to be done we have only to pay for it.

CHAPTER X

THE NEED FOR RESEARCH

*Present expenditure of public money on health serv-
ices and on research — Medical discoveries
have a monetary as well as a humanitarian
value — Present state of research — The
work of the fine-chemical firms — Secrecy
in research — A suggestion for the future.*

THERE are very few propositions about human needs that will receive assent from every-
body. Yet I think that no one will differ from the
view that it is better to be healthy than sick, and,
even in 1942, the great majority of mankind believes that it is better to be alive than dead. The
desire for life and health are more primitive and
basic than the wish for wealth or freedom; a citi-
zen should then insist that everything possible
should be done to ensure life and health to him
and his fellows. The only numerical measure of
desires is money — How much art thou sorry? In
England for example the State expends about
$125,000,000, and Local Governments about $150,-
000,000 on Health Services, while the contribu-
tions from National Health Insurance represented
another $150,000,000. Thus the nation's health

bill may be put at some $425,000,000.

An interesting anomaly at once appears — namely, that only a negligible proportion of this sum is expended on research. The greater part of the medical research done today is carried on at the great private hospitals; at the hospitals maintained by local authorities some clinical research is, of course, done, as it always will be where medical men are active. But the public expenditure on any research, which is not actually a part of the curing of patients, is extremely small.

Regarding the matter purely from a financial angle, sick people are an expensive luxury. Let us suppose that a new discovery shortens the period that pneumonia patients spend in hospital from five weeks to three weeks, and that twenty thousand such patients are treated in municipal hospitals each year. They certainly cost no less than $15 a week to maintain and treat, so the direct saving to the taxpayer and ratepayer is $1,800,000 per annum. Add to this the benefit payable to families while the breadwinner is incapacitated, and sickness, even considered with the cold eye of Mammon, seems to be well worth avoiding. If we capitalize that yearly saving at 5 per cent we may call the cash value of such discovery $120,000,000. I will not presume to set a price on lives actually saved. A hundred years ago a slave was worth about $400, equivalent to, let us say, $750 at the present value of the dollar. Presumably, a free citizen is worth no less and it is reasonable to suppose that a discovery such as the treatment of pneumonia with M & B 693, which can save twenty thousand lives yearly, is worth $15,000,000 per annum to the State. It is unpleasant to have to value lives in cash, but this is precisely what the nation has to do when it allocates its income to health services, education, defense, and the like.

Decrease in the sickness-rate or death-rate is obviously, from every point of view, one of the most desirable results that the State can bring about. Such a decrease can be brought about, first by improving wage-conditions and housing; secondly, by increasing medical services; thirdly, by medical research, on which the value of the others, in fact, depends. If every workman had earned $25 a week in 1840, it would not have prevented the people from dying like flies from cholera and typhoid, for these diseases abounded in every class of life until Pasteur and his followers showed us how they were transmitted. Nor, to-day, would a wage of $50 a week put a stop to the deaths from pneumonia or whooping-cough, and though it would certainly diminish the death-rate from tuberculosis it would not abolish it. Thus the increase in expenditure on medical treatment and improvement of conditions can only be a palliative of certain types of ill-health, whereas medical research holds out the promise, distant as it may be, of their total removal. Medical research is, indeed, the first necessity of health, for it shows what measures of prevention and cure can be applied.

We are very loath to pay anyone to do research. The contract between the rewards of private practice and of research is gigantic. Professorships are usually worth $5,000 to $7,500 per annum, lectureships and readerships $1,500 to $2,500; the men who obtain such posts might well earn three times that sum in private medical practice. Public bodies, such as hospitals and universities, give our men of science posts as lecturers, hospital physicians and surgeons, professors, heads of research departments, and, in fact, do their best to divert them from research by setting them to teach and organize. In the great majority of such posts, the first duty of their holders is to treat patients, and, in consequence, such medical research as can be done in the hospital ward receives the fullest attention, while work that requires to be done in the laboratory is, comparatively speaking, neglected. Hundreds of physicians can and will try out a new drug on human beings, but very little public provision is made for the research which leads to the synthesis of such drugs and their preliminary testing. The hospitals have in most cases a chemical department, but it is rather a means of teaching some elementary chemistry to unwilling medical students than an institution capable of carrying on extensive chemical researches. Universities have chemical departments where such researches could be carried on, but in the majority of cases there is no co-operation between their chemical workers and their biologists, let alone medical men. It is very rare for the university re-

search worker to take up the study of synthetic
drugs, for he has no certain means of securing the
co-operation of pathologists and practicing medical men.

The consequence of this lack of co-ordination
between the chemists and bacteriologists has been
the almost complete relinquishment of research in
chemotherapy to the great fine-chemical firms.
These are able to employ numerous chemists and
to direct their research to certain objects: they
can employ bacteriologists and pathologists to test
the drugs these chemists make. Is this not an ad-
mirable state of affairs? Certainly, if it be com-
pared with former conditions in which no such
researches were being carried out. Of the efficiency
of the present system there can indeed be no
doubt; the results obtained speak for it with no
uncertain voice. But a system which is efficient is
not necessarily perfect or beyond improvement,
and it is obviously desirable to consider how far
such work can be accelerated. One marvels at the
work which has been accomplished. Yet one must
murmur: *Cui bono?* For whose advantage are
these firms working? There can only be one
answer—their legal duty is to operate for the benefit of their shareholders. The question then arises
whether the interests of humanity at large and the
shareholder of the fine-chemical firm coincide. To
a very great extent they do. It is to the interest of
both that the firm should produce as many and as
efficient drugs as is possible. But this coincidence
is not complete. It is to the interest of humanity

that Messrs. B should produce new drugs and that
the world at large should use them, but it is to the
interest of Messrs. A that they should not; moreover, it is the commercial duty of the chemical
firms to make as much money as they can out of the
sale of a drug, but to the interest of humanity that
they should make as little as possible.

The first undesirable feature of the present system is competition on research.   The purest ethics
of science demand publication of results at the
earliest moment, so that other workers may be
aided in the pursuit of truth.   In fact, of course,
men of science are not saints, even though they are
not quite so predatory as the members of some
other professions.   They do not work entirely for
the pure crown of knowledge; they also work for
fame and promotion.   But the credit for a new discovery goes to the first man to announce it; so important results are usually announced very soon,
and often before the details of an investigation
have been completed.   The object of Messrs. A,
on the contrary, is not the reputation of being the
discoverers of the first member of a famous group
of drugs.   Their object is to be the only firm which
can market the drugs which the medical profession wish to buy.   They must, therefore, patent
their chemists' discoveries (which cannot be done
if details have been published) and must give as
few hints as possible to the research chemist of
their rivals.   So when Messrs. A find that a certain
drug has a certain power, they do not make this
public.   Their own employees, bound to secrecy,

work on it for months or even years until they have explored every possibility that the whole group of similar drugs may possibly present; they then take out patents, often phrased in the widest and vaguest terms; thus intending to gain protection for their discovery without giving more information than they need.   This secrecy is, of course, prejudicial to progress.   It prevents research workers from profiting by each other's conclusions — always a fertile source of inspiration. Moreover, it tends to the unnecessary duplication of labors, for two or even more teams of workers may investigate the same problem at the same time in ignorance of each other's efforts.

But *the work is done,* which is more than would happen if it were left to the hospitals and universities as at present constituted.

The second undesirable feature of commercial research comes to light when we ask: 'Who pays for it?'   Clearly the cost of research is met by the profits of the sale of drugs, which means that it is paid for by the sick and not the healthy.   Yet it is the latter that benefit in many respects, e.g. by the decrease of cost of health services, by diminished risk of infection, etc.   It is extremely desirable to keep the cost of drugs low, for in many communities this must make the difference between their use or disuse.   It would be, then, very desirable if they could be sold at the cost of manufacture, with, of course, the usual profit added thereto; and that they should not have to carry the additional cost of research.   I do not suggest that the price charged for drugs is, in fact, unreasonable; but the fact remains that there is no reason why it should not be so. If a sound patent for a drug is obtainable, the firm then manufactures the drug, without competition from its rivals, and sells it at the price which will yield the best monetary return. This may not be an unreasonably high price, but there is no reason why it should not be so, except considerations of humanity, or the hope of an increased sale. Humanitarian reasons cannot be relied upon, as was well shown by the manner in which the price of radium, used almost entirely for cancer treatment, was, in recent years, artificially inflated.

I would, therefore, suggest two ways of furthering the progress of chemotherapy. The first would be a great augmentation of chemo-therapeutic research, paid for by public money in the lively hope of a manifold saving on health services. Secondly, the refusal to grant patents for the manufacture of drugs. The two suggestions are quite independent. The former is immediately practicable; the other would be more difficult, perhaps impracticable, since patents are commonly international in scope.

As a means of furthering research in the subject, I would suggest that to every teaching hospital in the country there should be attached an Institute of Chemotherapy, properly and sufficiently endowed. Better results would be obtained from a number of smaller institutions, each under its own research director, than from a single mammoth institution, where personal contact and interchange of ideas between workers might be lacking. At each site there would then be the complete equipment of chemists, pathologists, bacteriologists, physicians — and patients. All work would be published at recent intervals. Patents would not in general be taken out, though in the case of a material whose manufacture should not be undertaken by any commercial firm the State might hold the patents, and assign the rights to suitable firms on condition that a reasonable price for the product should be fixed.

Could we afford to do this? I will say nothing about what we can afford in the midst of war, but I will confidently assert that a year ago we could have afforded such a scheme, and that it would, over a period of years, pay us handsomely. And, if it paid us not at all, except in the relief of suffering, I would maintain that we could afford it still. For each new thing discovered is not the possession only of us, here in our country and now in 1942, but of the whole population of the world, now and for as many years as shall pass until something better still be brought to light by the research workers of the future. Quinine has been relieving suffering for three hundred years, chloroform for ninety-three, diphtheria antitoxin for forty-five. Who can estimate the value of these things to the men of yesterday and today? How can we express our thanks better than by providing such things for men to come?

SULPHONAMIDE DRUGS (1940)

OFFICIAL OR USUAL TITLE	CHEMICAL NAME	OTHER TRADE NAMES	CHEMICAL FORMULA ATOM-SKELETON OF SULPHONAMIDE GROUP IN HEAVY TYPE
SULPHANILAMIDE (Made by most Firms)	PARA-AMINOBENZENE-SULPHONAMIDE	These are Legion see footnote below	
SULPHAPYRIDINE (May & Baker)	2-(PARA-AMINOBENZENE SULPHAMIDO) PYRIDINE	M&B. 693 DAGENAN	
PRONTOSIL RUBRUM (Bayer)	4'SULPHONAMIDO-2:4-DIA-MINO-AZOBENZENE	PRONTOSIL	
PRONTOSIL SOLUBLE (Bayer)	4'SULPHONAMIDOPHENYL-2-AZO-1-HYDROXY-7-ACETYLAMINONAPHTHALENE-3-6-DISULPHONIC ACID	PRONTOSIL PRONTOSIL S PRONTOSIL II NEOPRONTOSIL BAYER 102 RUBIAZOL INJECTABLE STREPTOZON S	
ULERON (Bayer)	4-(4'AMINOBENZENE-SUL-PHONAMIDO)-BENZENESUL-PHODIMETHYLAMIDE	DISEPTAL A ULIRON D.B.90 D.B.373	
RUBIAZOL (Roussel)	4'SULPHONAMIDO-2:4-DIAMINO-6-CARBOXYAZO-BENZENE		

174

PROSEPTASINE (May & Baker)	PARA-BENZYLAMINOBEN-ZENESULPHONAMIDE	BENZYLSULPHANILIDE SEPRASINE M&B.125 SETAZINE 46 R.P.	
SOLUSEPTASINE (May & Baker)	DISODIUM-PARA-(Γ-PHENYL-PROPYLAMINO)-BENZENE-SULPHONAMIDE	M & B 157 40 R.P.	
ALBUCID (Schering)	PARA-AMINOBENZENE-SUL-PHONACETAMIDE		
RODILONE[2] (Specia)	DI-(PARA-ACETYLAMINO-PHENYL) SULPHINE	F 1399	
AMBESID SOLUBLE (Schering)	SODIUM SUCCINYLPARA-MINOBENZENE-SULPHON-AMIDE		

SULPHANILAMIDE HAS 33 TRADE NAMES:- AMBESID, ASTREPTINE, COLSULANYDE, DESEPTYL, ERGASEPTINE, ERYSIPAN, GOMBARDOL, LYSOCOCCINE, NEOCOCCYL, ORGASEPTINE, P.A B.S., PRONTOSIL ALBUM, PRONTYLIN, PROSEPTINE, PROSEPTOL, PYSOCCINE, RUBIAZOL-A SEPTAMIDE, SEPTOPLIX, STOPTON ALBUM, STRAMID, STREPTAZOL, STREPTOCIDE, STREPTOCLASE, STREPTOZONE, SULFAMIDYL, SULFANA, SULFANIL, P SULPHAMIDOANILINE, SULPHONAMIDE - P, SUPRON, THERAPOL,..

INDEX

INDEX

INDEX